BE HEALTHIER NOW

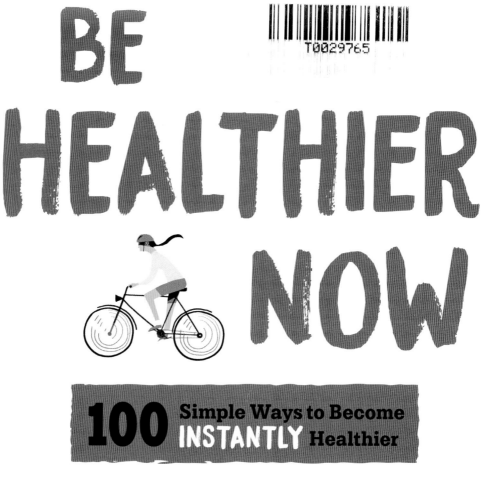

T0029765

100 Simple Ways to Become **INSTANTLY** Healthier

Written by **JACOB SAGER WEINSTEIN**

Illustrated by **FABIO SARDO**

odd dot

NEW YORK

For Rob Z. K. and Sheryl K. Z.

Now that somebody has dedicated a book on health and fitness to you, you're officially jocks. Sorry, but I don't make the rules.

Non est vivere, sed valere vita est.
Life isn't just being well. It's being well.
—Martial, circa AD 100

An imprint of Macmillan Children's Publishing Group, LLC
120 Broadway, New York, NY 10271 • OddDot.com
Odd Dot ® is a registered trademark of Macmillan Publishing Group, LLC

Joyful Books for Curious Minds

Text copyright © 2023 by Jacob Sager Weinstein
All rights reserved.

The Be Better Now Series is a trademark of Odd Dot.

WRITER Jacob Sager Weinstein
ILLUSTRATOR Fabio Sardo
DESIGNERS Caitlyn Hunter and Tim Hall
EDITOR Justin Krasner
VETTER Dr. Baturalp Baserdem

Library of Congress Cataloging-in-Publication Data is available.

ISBN 978-1-250-79508-3

Our books are available at special discounts when purchased in bulk for premiums and sales promotions as well as for fund-raising or educational use. Special editions or book excerpts also can be created to specification. For details, contact the Macmillan Corporate and Premium Sales Department at (800) 221-7945 ext. 5442, or send an email to MacmillanSpecialMarkets@macmillan.com.

First edition, 2023

Printed in China by Hung Hing Printing

10 9 8 7 6 5 4 3 2 1

CONTENTS

MOVE HEALTHY 43

EAT HEALTHY 79

HEALTHY ALL OVER 119

INTRODUCTION

Fitness is not the exclusive domain of the bronzed and the buff. It's your birthright as a human being. Whatever shape you're in, you can be healthier than you are, without making it your full-time job.

Be Healthier Now is a collection of 100 things you can do *today* to lead a healthier life. It includes tips on healthy eating and exercise, but it doesn't stop there. Fitness is about keeping every part of your body healthy and safe, from the top of your head to the tips of your toes.

I've tried to offer something new on every page. You might already know that sitting too long is bad for your health. But did you know that the cure for too much sitting could be something your grade school teacher told you *not* to do? See page 41.

Some tips will be about *what* you should do. On page 62, for example, I'll tell you how many steps a day you need to get for optimum health. (Contrary to what you've heard, it's *not* ten thousand.) Other tips will be about *how* you should do it. On page 63, I offer some tweaks you can make to your daily life to get those steps in.

Although this book has 100 healthy things you can do today, it doesn't have 100 things you *must* do today. You don't have to join a team *and* do a resistance band workout *and* quit a bad habit. Each step is meant to stand on its own. View *Be Healthier Now* as a menu of healthy possibilities rather than a series of ironclad mandates.

Now, I'm not a medical professional. I'm just an author who's interested in living a healthier life. If your health-care professionals disagree with any of my advice, then for heaven's sake . . . listen to them, not me! But I think you'll find they agree with most of what I have to say. I've based my advice on scientific studies and expert opinion. Researching this book has inspired me to lead a healthier, fitter life. I hope reading it does the same for you.

Read on—and be healthier NOW.

ICONS TO LOOK FOR:

Throughout this book, you'll notice a few recurring logos. Here's what they mean.

HABITS

Some of the things in this book are one-time lessons to learn. But many of them are habits you can implement, becoming a little healthier each time. The Habits logo will highlight these.

LEARN MORE

In writing this book, I read the work of people who know a lot more than I do. I've done my best to explain their work in a way that gives you concrete steps you can take right away. But inevitably, they've put more ideas in their books than I can present in one or two pages. If you want to read more, the Learn More logo will guide you to brilliant books that go further in depth.

HAPPINESS BONUS

I'm also the author of *Be Happier Now*. It turns out that a number of tips work equally well in either book. The Happiness Bonus logo will draw your attention to techniques that will make you simultaneously happier and healthier.

DON'T WORRY

Staying healthy shouldn't be scary! Look for the Don't Worry logo for some reassuring news.

THINK
HEALTHY

When it comes to good health, your brain is the most important organ in your body. Let's start off with some tips and techniques to get you in the right frame of mind.

HAVE A HEALTHY RELATIONSHIP WITH HEALTH

If you're reading this book, it's probably because you want to be healthier. That's great!

But sometimes that desire can get out of control. For people with eating disorders, body dysmorphia, or other issues around food and fitness, a book of health tips may not be the healthiest read.

It's important to me that *Be Healthier Now* makes your life better, not worse. So before you read on, check in with yourself to make sure you're in the right frame of mind to benefit from it.

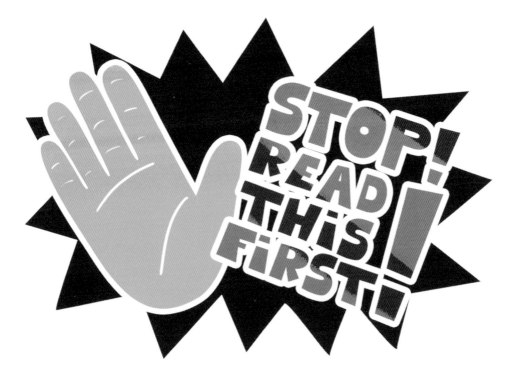

Symptoms of an Eating Disorder

If you have any of the following symptoms, **you may have an** eating disorder:

- You, or the people around you, are worried that you have an unhealthy relationship with food.
- You spend a lot of time worrying about your weight or body shape.
- You avoid social events if you think there will be food.
- You make yourself vomit or take laxatives after you eat.
- You have very strict food habits or routines.
- Your weight is very high or very low, given your age and height.

Symptoms of Body Dysmorphia

You may have body dysmorphia if your thoughts about your appearance:

- Cause you distress.
- Significantly interfere with your social life, education, work, or other aspects of your life.
- Affect your family or friends.
- Make you avoid many social situations.

STEP 1: If you recognize any of the symptoms listed above, or if you have a history of unhealthy behavior around food, fitness, or body image, turn the page for tips on finding professional help.

STEP 2: Once you've done that, put down this book until you're in a better place.

☐ If you've checked in with yourself to make sure you're approaching *Be Healthier Now* from a healthy place, give yourself the win.

TAKE MENTAL HEALTH PROBLEMS AS SERIOUSLY AS PHYSICAL PROBLEMS

Besides being worth treating purely for your own happiness, mental health problems have a raft of physical health consequences. Depression, for example, can cause heart disease, and heart disease can cause depression, leading to a dangerous downward spiral. You wouldn't try to cure heart disease on your own; don't struggle through mental health problems without professional help, either.

Signs You Might Benefit from Therapy

- You feel overwhelmingly helpless for an extended period.
- Things don't get better no matter what you try.
- You can't do your everyday tasks at work or home.
- You are constantly worried or anxious.
- You're navigating a particularly challenging life event.
- You have a chronic physical illness that's negatively affecting your emotional life.
- You're doing something that's harming you or the people around you.
- You just need a nonjudgmental ear to listen while you talk.

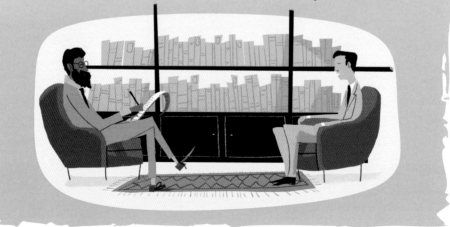

STEP 1: Do any of the signs on the previous page apply to you?

STEP 2: If so, it's worth checking in with a mental health professional. Some ways to find one:

- Ask a friend or family member for a recommendation.
- You can ask a nonmedical professional for suggestions, too. A divorce attorney might know somebody who can help you cope with divorce, for example.
- Get a referral through your doctor or insurance plan.
- Contact your local community health center, or the psychology department of a local university.
- Look up your local psychological association at apa.org/about/apa/organizations/associations
- Use the American Psychological Association's online locator: locator.apa.org

STEP 3: Book an appointment.

STEP 4: Show up for it.

STEP 5: After the appointment, reflect on how it went. If the therapist didn't feel like the right match, don't give up. You wouldn't give up on dating after a bad first date; don't stop seeking a psychotherapist after one bad session. When you find a therapist you connect with, it will be worth it.

☐ If you've had an appointment with a mental health professional— or even booked one—give yourself the win.

APPRECIATE THE BODY YOU HAVE

It's profitable to make you feel bad about your body. But ignore the people trying to sell you diet pills, fitness gizmos, and even (ahem) health books by convincing you there's something wrong with you.

Of course you can always be better than you are. If I didn't believe that, I wouldn't have written this book. But I also believe your goal should be a healthy body, not a trendy one.

STEP 1: Make a list of impressive things your body can do. Define "impressive" as broadly as possible, and don't forget to include things that most human bodies can do—if walking upright isn't an incredible accomplishment, why did it take evolution 3.8 billion years to figure it out?

STEP 2: Do something nice for your body, whether it's a massage, a long bath, or even a nap.

STEP 3: On the video website of your choice, search for "ideal body types throughout history" for an insight into how arbitrary body standards are.

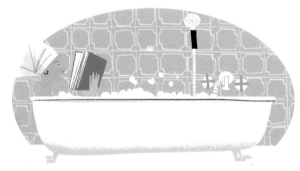

If you've appreciated the body you've got, appreciate the win.

REMEMBER THE WHY

Some of the tips in this book focus on *what* you should do (like get regular exercise). Many of them focus on *how* you should do it (like parking your car at the far end of the lot, page 63). But you'll find it easier to stick to the *what* and the *how* if you remember the *why*. Think about the people you're staying healthy for, and the good you can do if you're in good shape.

STEP 1: Think about somebody important to you. How can you make their life richer by being in better health? For that matter, how can you make their life richer just by being around longer?

STEP 2: Think about something you're looking forward to. How will you enjoy it more if you're fit and healthy?

STEP 3: Think of an ordinary day you felt healthy, and an ordinary day you didn't. How did being healthy make you happier?

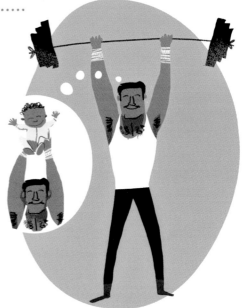

☐ If you've remembered one good reason to stay healthy, remember to check this box.

CONSUME HEALTH NEWS RESPONSIBLY

As medical news filters out into the world, it tends to get steadily more sensationalized. Fortunately, a few simple rules can help you separate the news from the nonsense.

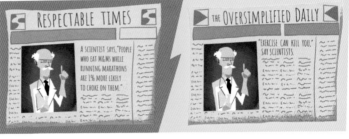

STEP 1: Trust a peer-reviewed medical journal over a respectable newspaper; a respectable newspaper over a tabloid; and a tabloid over a social media post.

STEP 2: Even the most responsible newspaper has to simplify a twenty-page research study to fit it into a few columns. Always assume that the original study was more cautious and nuanced than its media coverage suggests.

STEP 3: If you read a report today that contradicts something you read yesterday, it doesn't mean scientists can't make up their minds. Different reporters may have summarized the same report differently.

STEP 4: Watch out for reputation bleed, where somebody's nonmedical credentials earn attention for their crackpot medical theories. For example, Nobel Prize–winning chemist Linus Pauling insisted that vitamin C could cure cancer and mental illness, stubbornly ignoring the many studies that proved him wrong.

STEP 5: Above all, listen to your own doctor, who has spent years studying medicine and knows your specific medical history.

> ☐ If you got health news from a reliable source, or approached an unreliable source with skepticism, trust that you've won.

MEDITATE

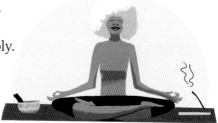

Meditation isn't new; people have been doing it for thousands of years. (Although not the same person. His legs would probably have cramped up by now.)

But the scientific study of meditation is new. Current evidence suggests that it can reduce your stress levels, help you sleep better, and lower your risk of heart disease.

STEP 1: Find a quiet place, and sit comfortably. You don't have to fold your legs into a pretzel (unless you want to).

STEP 2: Set a timer for a short and manageable time. If you've never meditated before, try it for as little as a minute and then increase it a bit for your next session.

STEP 3: Close your eyes.

STEP 4: Notice how your breath feels as it goes in and out. Feel your chest rise and fall. There's no need to pass judgment or draw any conclusions; just let yourself experience the sensations.

STEP 5: Let yourself become aware of your feet. Notice what sensations they're currently feeling. Again, don't judge—just notice. Slowly let your attention flow up your body, bit by bit, all the way to the top of your head.

STEP 6: If your mind wanders, that's perfectly natural. Just gently bring it back to what your body is experiencing.

STEP 7: Repeat Step 5 or 6 or both until the timer goes off.

☐ If you meditated for even a minute, meditate on your win.

BOX BREATHE

You might not think that yoga and Navy SEAL training have much in common, but they share at least one technique. It's called *sama vritti pranayama* or "box breathing," depending on whether you're wearing soft, comfortable clothing or camouflage. By either name, it can keep you calm in a stressful situation.

And staying calm can save your life, even if you're not about to infiltrate an enemy military base. Stress reduces your resistance to infection, and chronic stress is a major cause of cardiovascular disease.

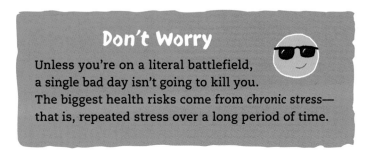

Don't Worry

Unless you're on a literal battlefield, a single bad day isn't going to kill you. The biggest health risks come from *chronic stress*—that is, repeated stress over a long period of time.

STEP 1: In a calm moment, set aside a few minutes to practice this breathing technique.

STEP 2: Exhale completely, mentally counting to four.

STEP 3: Pause for another count of four. Don't hold your breath frantically as if you are about to dive under water! Just gently wait before you breathe in again.

STEP 4: Breathe slowly in for another count of four.

STEP 5: Gently wait before breathing out for another count of four.

STEP 6: Repeat this for several cycles. It may help to imagine that each cycle is a trip around a box—hence the name.

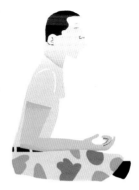

STEP 7: Next time you're in an intense situation, use the technique to help reduce the physiological effects of stress. As a bonus, you'll find it helps you think more clearly, too.

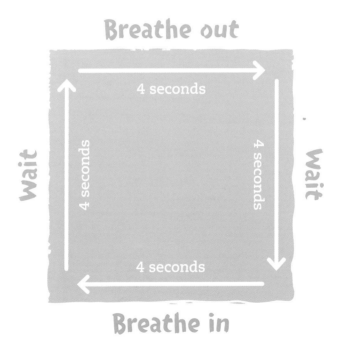

Breathe out

4 seconds

wait

4 seconds

4 seconds

wait

4 seconds

Breathe in

☐ If you've practiced a stress-reduction technique in a calm moment or used it in a stressful one, relax into the win.

TREAT HAPPINESS AS A MEDICAL NECESSITY

Numerous studies have found a link between positive emotions and overall health.

I admit: It's hard to know which direction that link goes. Are people healthy because they're happy? Or happy because they're healthy? My best guess is that it goes both ways. And if I'm wrong, and you pursue a happy life

To learn more, read my book *Be Happier Now.*

and then discover that it didn't help you stay healthy . . . well, you still ended up happy. As worst-case scenarios go, that's a pretty darn good one.

Of all the tips in this book, this one might seem the most redundant. Who needs to be told to pursue happiness? Alas, the answer turns out to be most of us. We'll put aside our responsibilities if we have a heart attack—but not for the small happiness interventions that might prevent one.

STEP 1: Find something that makes you happy, whether it's embracing the love of your life in a lush field of roses or doing a crossword.

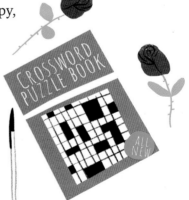

STEP 2: Make time for it in your day.

STEP 3: If it feels indulgent, ask yourself: Wouldn't you make time for a medical necessity?

☐ If you've taken one step to leading a happy life, view that as a psychological *and* physiological win.

A SLEEP-FRIENDLY BRAIN

Besides setting up your bedroom for a good night's sleep (page 26), it's important to set up your mind, too.

STEP 1: Turn off your electronic devices at least thirty minutes before bedtime.

STEP 2: Establish some relaxing rituals to cue your brain to sleep. Reading in bed, taking a warm bath, or doing gentle yoga are all good possibilities.

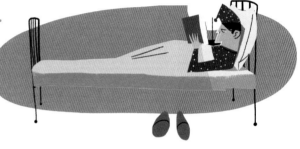

STEP 3: If you often find your mind racing when you get into bed, preempt the race by choosing a calm and relaxing mental picture, such as a peaceful meadow. When you turn out the lights, imagine the picture in as much sensory detail as you can. If you notice your attention wandering, gently bring it back to the image.

STEP 4: Go to bed and get up at roughly the same times every day. Luxurious though it feels to sleep in on weekends, it can make Monday mornings even harder.

STEP 5: If you aren't asleep after twenty minutes, get up and do something relaxing without exposing yourself to too much artificial light. When you start to feel sleepy, try again.

If you've taken steps to prepare your mind for sleep, you can drift off to thoughts of victory.

THE MIND DIET

Bad news: If you make it to your seventies, there's a 5 percent chance you'll suffer from dementia. By the time you're in your nineties, the odds rise to 37.4 percent.

Good news: You can do things now to help you end up on the right side of those odds. Your brain is part of your body, and almost anything you do to keep your body healthy will also protect your brain. (See page 16 for the exceptions.)

When it comes to healthy eating, one diet in particular seems to protect against dementia. Following it strictly is associated with a 53 percent lower chance of getting Alzheimer's. And if you can't stick to it rigorously, that's okay. Even following the MIND diet moderately well is associated with a 35 percent lower risk.

STEP 1: Eat at least some foods listed on the opposite page.

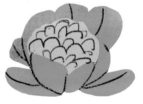

....

STEP 2: Don't eat more than one tablespoon of butter or margarine a day. Don't eat more than one serving of red meat, pastry, sweets, fried food, or fast food per week.

....

STEP 3: If you can't stick rigorously to Steps 1 and 2, just try to eat more of the stuff you're supposed to eat and less of the stuff you aren't.

The MIND Diet

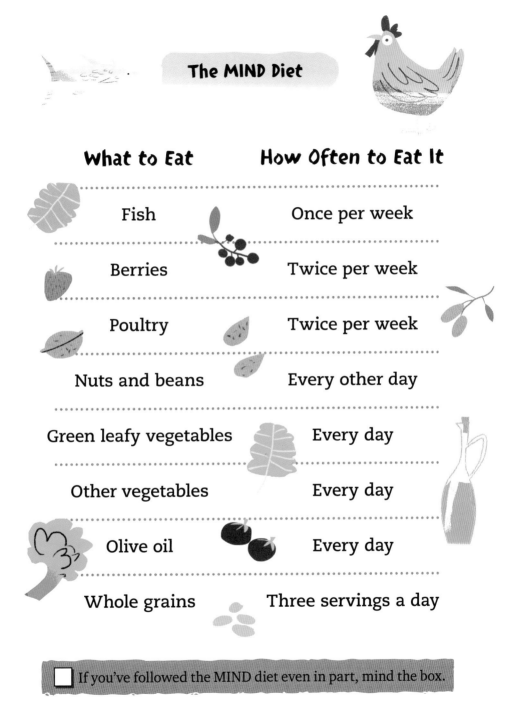

What to Eat	How Often to Eat It
Fish	Once per week
Berries	Twice per week
Poultry	Twice per week
Nuts and beans	Every other day
Green leafy vegetables	Every day
Other vegetables	Every day
Olive oil	Every day
Whole grains	Three servings a day

☐ If you've followed the MIND diet even in part, mind the box.

DON'T SCORE ON YOUR OWN BRAIN

Like any form of exercise, riding a bike helps keep your brain healthy—except when you smash your skull into the pavement. That happens more often than you might imagine; two-thirds of hospital admissions after bike accidents are the result of head injury.

Similarly, sports are great for your cardiovascular system, which does all kinds of good things for your brain . . . until you deliberately smash your skull into a soccer ball or another human being. Soccer players who frequently head balls do worse on tests of memory and verbal ability. Football players, boxers, and hockey players may be at greater risk of Alzheimer's and chronic traumatic encephalopathy.

However you keep moving, make sure your brain stays protected.

STEP 1: If you ride a wheeled vehicle without a top—anything from a skateboard to a motorcycle—go to a store that sells appropriate head protection.

STEP 2: Let one of the salespeople help you find a properly fitting helmet. While you're at it, ask them to show you how to wear it properly.

STEP 3: If you play a sport that involves smashing your head into something, switch to a sport that's less traumatic for your brain. If you simply can't give it up, shield your skull as thoroughly as your sport allows.

☐ If you've protected your brain while exercising or doing a sport, score!

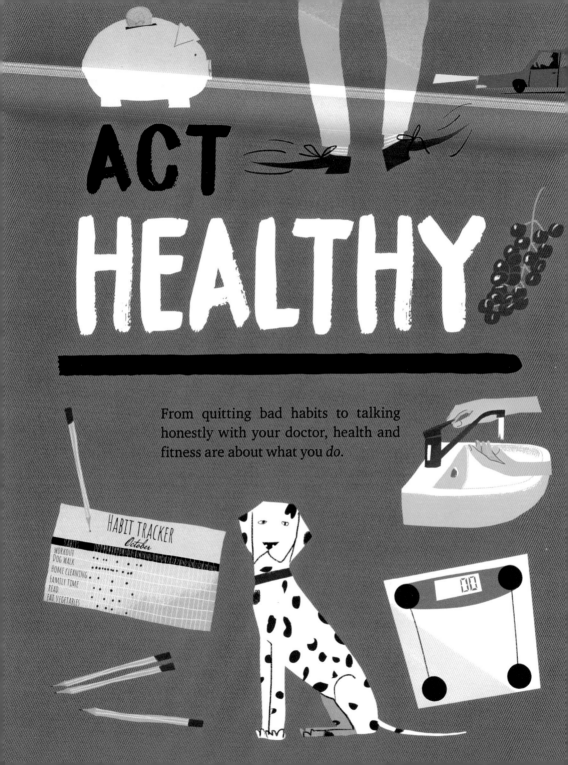

ACT HEALTHY

From quitting bad habits to talking honestly with your doctor, health and fitness are about what you *do*.

HABIT TRACKER
October

HABITS
WORKOUT
DOG WALK
HOME CLEANING
FAMILY TIME
READ
EAT VEGETABLES

00

DRIVE SAFELY

Let's give thanks to the health-care professionals in our lives: our doctors, our nurses, our driving instructors.

Surprised by that last one? Don't be. Driving is one of the riskiest common activities around, and the vast majority of accidents are caused by driver behavior.

If you're reading this in the US, you're at an especially high risk. Americans are more likely to die in a crash than Brits, Swedes, Aussies, Danes, or Canadians. If America could bring its rate of accidents down to the level of those countries, it would save eighteen thousand lives a year.

You probably think you're already driving safely. In one survey, 93 percent of Americans thought they were better drivers than average. You don't have to be a mathematician to know they can't all be right.

Basic Safety

IF EVERY AMERICAN DOES THIS...	...IT WILL SAVE THIS MANY LIVES PER YEAR
Properly use seat belts, booster seats, and car seats	**9,500**
Don't drive drunk	**10,500**
Drive at the speed limit	**9,500**

STEP 1: Buckle up when you get into the car, no matter how short a trip it is. Make sure any children in the car are in properly installed car seats and booster seats.

....

STEP 2: Drive at the speed limit.

....

STEP 3: Before you take your first drink of the evening, have a plan for how you'll get home without driving.

....

STEP 4: No matter how long you've been driving and how good a driver you think you are, consider taking a refresher course. Ask the instructor to help identify and correct any bad habits you've picked up in your years on the road.

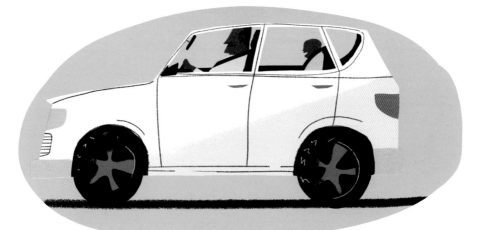

☐ If you've taken steps to improve your driving safety, take a victory lap.

GET IN THE HABIT

Turning a healthy action into a healthy habit will bring you a lifetime of benefits. How long it takes to reach that point depends on the person and the habit. One study found it took an average of sixty-six days, although it can be as little as eighteen or as many as 254.

 To learn more, read *The Power of Habit* by Charles Duhigg.

You can get there through a cycle of *trigger, action,* and *reward.*

STEP 1: Identify a healthy activity you want to make into a habit. Let's say it's laying out your workout clothes in advance (page 57).

STEP 2: Choose a trigger. Make it a concrete thing you already do regularly, like brushing your teeth before you shower. It could even be a preexisting bad habit: "I can't check Twitter until I've laid out my workout clothes." This is called **temptation bundling**.

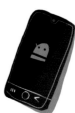

STEP 3: Identify a reward you get from your new habit. There might be a built-in reward, like the pride you feel in setting yourself up for exercise success. If not, you can create one. Just make sure you're not creating a new unhealthy habit. Smelling the mint in your window garden is a good reward. Eating an entire pint of mint chocolate chip ice cream? Not so good.

STEP 4: Do your desired action as soon as the trigger occurs.

STEP 5: Enjoy the reward.

STEP 6: For an extra motivation boost, consider tracking your healthy habits. Even the small gesture of making a check mark can be its own reward. You can use a fancy computer app, or draw your own tracker with crayons on scrap paper . . . or use the built-in tracker on the inside jacket of this very book.

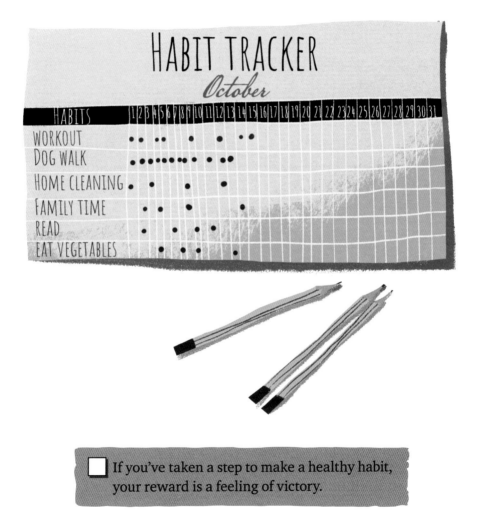

HABIT TRACKER
October

HABITS	1	2	3	4	5	6	7	8	9	10	11	12	13	14	15	16	17	18	19	20	21	22	23	24	25	26	27	28	29	30	31
WORKOUT	•			•	•			•				•		•		•	•														
DOG WALK	•	•	•	•	•	•	•	•	•	•		•		•		•	•														
HOME CLEANING	•		•				•				•			•																	
FAMILY TIME		•		•			•				•				•																
READ		•				•		•			•																				
EAT VEGETABLES			•		•		•		•			•																			

☐ If you've taken a step to make a healthy habit, your reward is a feeling of victory.

GET OUT OF THE HABIT

Making healthy habits is half the battle. The other half? Losing unhealthy ones.

Note that this technique works for psychological habits. Addictions that are both physical and psychological (like tobacco) may require consulting with a medical professional.

STEP 1: Identify a habit you want to break.

STEP 2: Notice what triggers it. Do you walk over and grab a handful of chocolate chips whenever you get stuck in the book you're writing? (That happened to, um, a friend of mine.)

STEP 3: Identify the rewards you get from the action and figure out a way to substitute for them. My . . . friend . . . realized he got a change of scenery, a quick break, and a sweet taste.

STEP 4: Find an alternative, healthier way to get those rewards—and make it easier than the unhealthy habit you want to break. My friend put the chocolate chips up high and started leaving a container of washed grapes right on my kitchen counter. I mean, his counter. (Aw, heck. It was me.)

STEP 5: Next time the trigger creates the urge, indulge in the healthier alternative. The first few times, it will take active willpower. Eventually, you'll find it becoming automatic.

> ☐ If you've worked toward breaking a bad habit, reward yourself with a victory.

QUIT IT

If you smoke, you probably already know it's bad for you. Smoking is the leading cause of preventable death in America, which is probably why 68 percent of smokers want to quit. Many of them have succeeded: At this point, there are more ex-smokers than smokers.

If you want to join that throng of successful quitters, I believe in you! It's a frustratingly hard habit to break—but there are ways to make it easier.

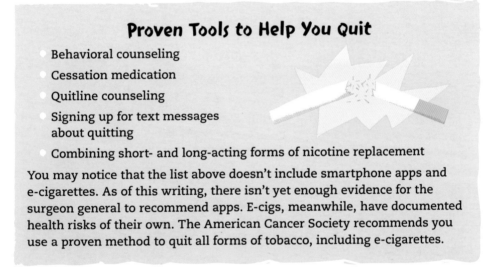

Proven Tools to Help You Quit

- Behavioral counseling
- Cessation medication
- Quitline counseling
- Signing up for text messages about quitting
- Combining short- and long-acting forms of nicotine replacement

You may notice that the list above doesn't include smartphone apps and e-cigarettes. As of this writing, there isn't yet enough evidence for the surgeon general to recommend apps. E-cigs, meanwhile, have documented health risks of their own. The American Cancer Society recommends you use a proven method to quit all forms of tobacco, including e-cigarettes.

STEP 1: Tell your doctor you want to quit, and ask for their advice. Even a brief consultation with a doctor increases your odds of successfully quitting.

STEP 2: Seek out one or more of the proven treatments above. Every one has convincing scientific evidence that it helps smokers quit. Combining multiple techniques may make them even more effective.

☐ If you've taken one step to quit smoking (or if you've already quit, or just never started), take a deep breath of victory.

WORK LESS, LIVE LONGER

If you've ever felt like long work hours were sapping your life force, science has your back. In study after study, overwork has been linked to heart disease and alcoholism, and it may even cause cognitive decline.

And what do businesses get in exchange for killing their employees? Lower profits. Well-rested workplaces are more productive ones. There's a vast body of research documenting that people who routinely work more than sixty hours per week accomplish *less* than those who work fewer than fifty.

STEP 1: If you're in a position of authority, make your workplace happier, healthier, and more productive by keeping hours below fifty per week. If you're already below fifty hours, try going below forty. You may find your employees get more done.

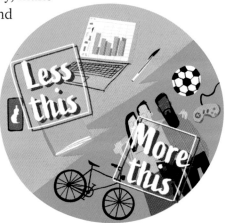

STEP 2: If your workplace offers time off or any other benefits that will make your life less stressful, take full advantage of them.

STEP 3: If you can choose where to work, pay close attention to the working hours of your potential workplace.

STEP 4: If you can't avoid long hours, seek out de-stressing activities in whatever free time you've got. Meditation (page 9) and the seven-minute workout (page 70) can offer major mood boosts in short bursts of time.

☐ If you've taken steps to make your workplace less stressful, you've worked up a win.

DETECT TROUBLE

If you want to make a firefighter's life easier, install a pole, a fire truck, and a dalmatian in your home.

Or you could just get a smoke detector. It's not as cute as a dalmatian, but it's less likely to pee on your carpet.

Don't Worry

Most smoke and carbon monoxide detectors live their entire lives without detecting any real emergencies.

STEP 1: Buy a reliable brand of smoke detector from a store you trust. This is not a place to cut corners.

STEP 2: Now get more smoke detectors. The US Fire Administration recommends you put them inside and outside each bedroom or sleeping area, with at least one on every level of your home.

STEP 3: Smoke alarms should be replaced ten years after they were made. Check the manufacture date of every smoke alarm you've got, and put a reminder on your calendar or phone to replace it.

STEP 4: While you're at it, set up a monthly reminder to check the batteries.

STEP 5: If you have a gas water heater, a wood-burning furnace, or any other nonelectric source of heat, get a carbon monoxide detector, too. Carbon monoxide is an invisible, odorless gas that can cause dizziness, headaches, and even death.

STEP 6: Carbon monoxide doesn't respect property boundaries. If you share walls or floors with another home, get a carbon monoxide detector even if you yourself have only electric heat.

☐ If you've purchased or maintained a smoke or carbon monoxide detector, give yourself the win.

A SLEEP-FRIENDLY BEDROOM

A good night's sleep is a cornerstone of good health. And the right bedroom environment is a cornerstone of a good night's sleep.

With a few simple steps, you can set yourself up for a good night's rest—and a good next day.

STEP 1: Don't do anything stressful in your bedroom, whether it's answering work emails or doomscrolling social media. You want your mind to associate your bedroom with relaxation.

STEP 2: Don't use your bed for anything other than sleep, relaxing reading, or physical intimacy.

STEP 3: The American Academy of Sleep Medicine recommends a bedroom temperature of around sixty-eight degrees Fahrenheit. Some doctors recommend a range from sixty to sixty-five degrees. The takeaway: Individuals vary, so you may need to experiment. The temperature that best helps you sleep may feel cold when you're outside the covers.

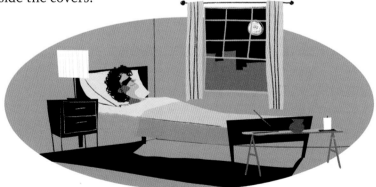

☐ If you've taken steps to make your bedroom a happy sleep environment, you can rest on your laurels.

MIND THE GAP

When you're angry, it's hard to imagine being calm. When you're full, it's hard to imagine being hungry.

Psychologists call this the **hot-cold empathy gap**. If you've ever bought a bag of fun-size candy in the sincere belief that you would eat it over a month, and then found yourself finishing it in twenty-four hours, you have experienced the gap.

The hot-cold empathy gap is a part of human nature, and you can't overcome it completely—but knowing it exists will help you predict your own behavior more accurately.

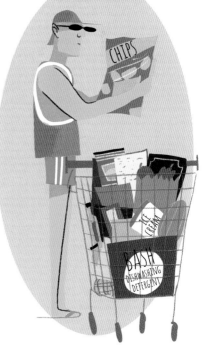

STEP 1: If you plan to bring unhealthy food into your house, on the theory that you can have small amounts of it and then stop, review what happened when you last tried something similar. Were you able to have reasonable amounts? If not, what makes you think this time will be different?

STEP 2: Review your plans when you're hungry. This will help you predict more accurately how many chips you'll actually eat when they're sitting in front of you and your mouth is watering.

☐ If you've planned with the hot-cold empathy gap in mind, warmly congratulate yourself.

MAKE A LIST AND CHECK IT TWICE

Nobody knows more about your health than you—but in an emergency, you might not be conscious to share your knowledge. And even when you're at the top of your game, you might struggle to remember your physician's phone number or the exact details of your prescriptions. Putting it all in one place could save your life and can certainly save you time and stress.

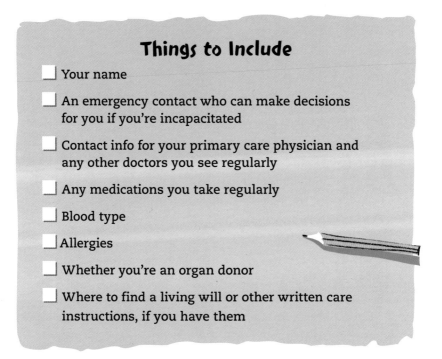

Things to Include

- [ ] Your name
- [ ] An emergency contact who can make decisions for you if you're incapacitated
- [ ] Contact info for your primary care physician and any other doctors you see regularly
- [ ] Any medications you take regularly
- [ ] Blood type
- [ ] Allergies
- [ ] Whether you're an organ donor
- [ ] Where to find a living will or other written care instructions, if you have them

STEP 1: Write down every piece of relevant health information you can think of.

. . . .

STEP 2: Save it as a computer file with a clear document name, like "Nick's Emergency Health Information."

STEP 3: Print out a copy and keep it in your wallet.

STEP 4: Make sure the important people in your life know where to find it.

STEP 5: If you carry a smartphone, search for the emergency screen setting. This will let you choose what medical information is visible to somebody who has access to your phone but doesn't know the password.

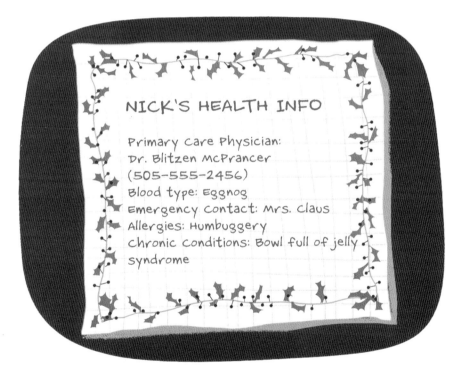

NICK'S HEALTH INFO

Primary Care Physician:
Dr. Blitzen McPrancer
(505-555-2456)
Blood type: Eggnog
Emergency Contact: Mrs. Claus
Allergies: Humbuggery
Chronic Conditions: Bowl full of jelly syndrome

☐ If you've made a list of important health information, list it as one of your wins.

SNEEZE INTO YOUR ELBOW

Most of the tips in this book will keep you healthy. This one will keep everybody around you healthy. Cover your mouth when you cough or sneeze, especially if you're not wearing a mask. By using your elbow, you avoid getting germs on your hand and transmitting them to every door-knob you open.

STEP 1: If you feel a cough or sneeze coming on, hold the crook of your elbow up to your mouth.

STEP 2: Sneeze or cough into it, thereby saving everybody around you from inhaling your germs.

STEP 3: Accept high fives with your pristine hands.

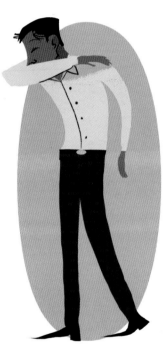

☐ If you've sneezed or coughed into your elbow, use your nice, clean fingers to pat your back.

SAY NO TO YOUR DOCTOR

In writing this book, I asked some health-care professionals what they wished people would do for their own health. Many of the answers were things I would have predicted, like "Stop Drinking Sugar" (page 99) and "Get Vaxxed" (page 38). But one answer caught me completely off guard.

What follows is not based on any scientific study. It's one primary care physician's advice. But once I got over my surprise, it made perfect sense to me, and I think it's well worth including.

STEP 1: If your doctor offers advice that you know you won't take, don't pretend that you will. Firmly say, "No, I won't take that medicine" or "No, I'm not going to give up eating mousetraps" or whatever the case may be.

. . . .

STEP 2: Ask your doctor what the next best option is. Work with them to find advice that you will actually take.

. . . .

STEP 3: You may end up with an equally good option. And even if you end up with something the doctor doesn't think is as good ("Eat mousetraps, but at least take the mouse out first"), it will still be a step forward.

. . . .

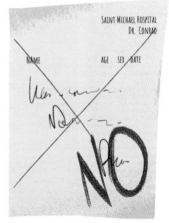

STEP 4: Similarly, if you get home and realize you're not going to take the advice or the medicine . . . or if you start taking it and then decide to stop . . . let your doctor know and work with them to find a replacement.

☐ If you've been honest with your doctor about your preferences, you've earned a win.

GIVE YOURSELF A CASH REWARD

When I was in college, my roommates and I found ourselves skipping more classes than we should have. So we made a pact: Every time one of us missed a class, we'd put twenty-five cents in a jar. At the end of the term, whoever missed the fewest classes would get the whole jar.

Miraculously, it worked. The expense of a college education and the potential future rewards for doing well didn't get us out of bed for a 9 AM class. Putting one darn quarter into a jar did.

Our behavior wasn't rational—but it may be universal. A megastudy of 61,293 gym members showed that offering a bonus of just nine cents for returning to the gym after a missed workout was the single most effective way of helping people stick with an exercise routine.

STEP 1: Identify a healthy habit you want to maintain.

STEP 2: Find a paying accountability buddy—somebody who is willing to donate a buck or two to your efforts.

STEP 3: Agree that if you miss your habit more than once in a row, you'll give them some token amount. And if you succeed in maintaining your habit a certain number of times in a row, they'll give you a token amount.

☐ If you've found a paying accountability buddy, or stuck with a habit because you've got one, deposit a victory into your account.

BUZZ OFF

Consider the common mosquito. Bill Gates (who knows a thing or two about bugs) once called it "the most dangerous animal on earth." He makes a convincing case: Besides being irritating little pests, they can carry dengue fever, encephalitis, West Nile virus, and a whole host of other nasties. Add it all up, and mosquitoes kill more people every year than sharks, wolves, bears, and lions combined.

Don't Worry Most mosquitoes are just nuisances. They're far more likely to annoy you than kill you.

Here are some mosquito bite prevention tips that could save your life (and will definitely save your sanity).

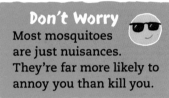

STEP 1: If you're going to be in an area with mosquito-borne illnesses, make sure you're up to date on the right vaccinations.

STEP 2: Use an EPA-registered insect repellent like DEET or oil of lemon eucalyptus. If you're putting it on kids, check the label first to make sure it's suitable.

STEP 3: If you're wearing sunscreen, put on the sunscreen first, and the repellent after.

STEP 4: Cover strollers and baby carriers with mosquito netting.

STEP 5: If you get a mosquito bite, don't scratch it. I know, I know—this is easier advice to give than to follow. But scratching increases your risk of infection. Try putting an ice pack over the bite for ten minutes to make it itch less or buy anti-itch cream. You can also take one tablespoon of baking soda, add just enough water to form a paste (about one teaspoon); and leave it on the itch for ten minutes before washing it off.

☐ If you've taken one step to protect yourself from mosquitoes, feel the victory buzz.

WASH YOUR HANDS

In the war against disease, some weapons are the modern result of multi-billion-dollar investments. And some are ancient and cheap. In the latter category: soap.

It doesn't even have to be fancy antibacterial soap. Pretty much any soap you buy will contain *surfactants,* compounds that can pry open germs, trap the biomaterials inside, and carry them down the drain.

If you've heard the advice to keep scrubbing for twenty seconds and wondered whether there was any science behind it: There is. That's about how long it takes the soap's surfactants to do their job across the entire complex and wrinkly surface of your hand.

STEP 1: Wet your hands with clean, running water. Turn off the tap, and apply soap. (If you don't have soap, it's still worth washing with water alone—that will get rid of some germs, although nowhere near as many.)

STEP 2: Lather your entire hands—the backs, the fronts, the fingers, the spaces between the fingers, and your web shooters. (That last one may apply only to certain incarnations of Spider-Man.) Be vigorous—keeping the soap moving forcefully helps it do its job.

STEP 3: Keep scrubbing for at least twenty seconds. That's roughly the time it takes to sing "Happy Birthday" twice.

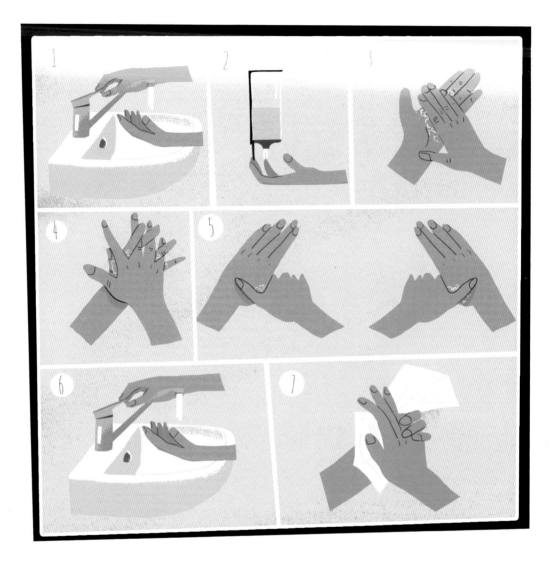

☐ If you've washed your hands properly, you just cleaned up.

MONITOR YOUR WEIGHT (BUT MONITOR YOUR MONITORING)

Research shows that people who monitor their weight regularly are more likely to shed it.

But there's an important caveat: People who suffer from an eating disorder (page 2) may be better off ignoring the scales entirely.

STEP 1: If you have symptoms of an eating disorder, find a mental health professional who can help you get better (page 4).

STEP 2: If you're confident you have a healthy relationship with food but you would be healthier at a lower weight, get a scale.

STEP 3: Weigh yourself at least once a week. You can track the results with a pen and paper or a fancy Wi-Fi scale—the method doesn't matter.

STEP 4: Remember that weight naturally fluctuates daily, depending on how hydrated you are, when you last used the toilet, and many other factors. Don't worry too much about day-to-day fluctuations.

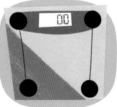

STEP 5: Keep an eye out for long-term trends. If you notice your weight steadily creeping toward an unhealthy high or low, consider whether you can adapt healthier eating habits.

STEP 6: Consider supplementing your weight measurements with body fat or waist circumference (page 37).

☐ If you've monitored your weight (and your attitude toward food) today, track your progress by checking the box.

KEEP AN EYE ON YOUR WAISTLINE

Your scale can help you monitor fluctuations in your weight—but weight itself is only a loose proxy for health. Ten extra pounds of muscle is a good thing; ten extra pounds of fat is not. And fat can be more risky in certain places—belly fat is more closely associated with health risks than fat elsewhere.

As with all body measurements, skip this one if you have concerns about your relationship with food (page 2).

STEP 1: Get a tape measure and put it around your waist halfway between your hips and your rib cage, just above the level of your belly button. The tape should be tight but not digging into your skin.

STEP 2: Breath out naturally and take the measurement.

STEP 3: As a rough guide, your waist diameter should be about half your height. Above that, and you increase your risk of heart problems and other medical conditions. If you need to lose some inches, see the Eat Healthy section (page 79).

STEP 4: Feel free to treat your waist diameter as a one-time measurement. Or record it on paper or with an app and track it over time. (Remember, it will naturally fluctuate from day to day; you're only looking for long-term trends.)

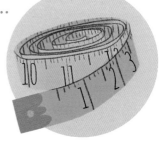

☐ If you've measured your waistline once, give yourself the win.

GET VAXXED

Some human inventions are mixed blessings, like the internal combustion engine and social media. But vaccines are an unequivocal good—unless you're a germ. By one estimate, they save two million to three million lives *every single year.*

By getting vaxxed, you're not just protecting yourself. You're helping save the lives of your fellow citizens who are immunocompromised or otherwise unable to benefit from vaccines. Getting vaccinated is like getting a bulletproof vest while simultaneously dragging somebody out of a burning building. As soon as they invent a vaccine against mixed metaphors, I'm getting that one, too.

STEP 1: If you're comfortable with medical details, consult the chart to see whether you've missed any vaccinations. Otherwise, just check in with your doctor to make sure you're up to date.

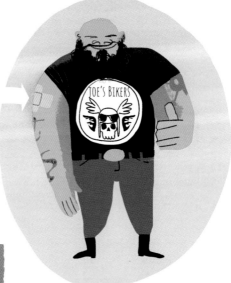

STEP 2: Make sure any kids you're responsible for are up to date on their shots as well.

☐ If you're up to date on your vaccinations, inject some victory.

Vaccines Recommended by Age

VACCINE	AGES 19–26	27–49	50–64	65+
Influenza inactivated (IIV4) or Influenza recombinant (RIV4)	1 dose annually			
	OR			
Influenza live attenuated (LAIV4)	1 dose annually			
Tetanus, diphtheria, pertussis (Tdap or Td)	1 dose Tdap each pregnancy; 1 dose Td/Tdap for wound managment			
	1 dose Tdap, then 1 dose Td or Tdap booster every 10 years			
Measles, mumps, rubella (MMR)	1 or 2 doses depending on indication (if born in 1957 or later)			
Varicella (VAR)	2 doses (if born in 1980 or later)		2 doses	
Zoster recombinant (RZV)	2 doses for immunocompromising conditions		2 doses	
Human papillomavirus (HPV)	2 or 3 doses depending on age at initial vaccination or condition	ages 27–45		
Pneumococcal (PCV15, PCV20, PPSV23)	1 dose PCV15 followed by PPSV23 OR 1 dose PCV20			1 dose PCV15 followed by PPSV23 OR 1 dose PCV20
Hepatitis A (HepA)	2 or 3 doses depending on vaccine			
Hepatitis B (HepB)	2, 3, or 4 doses depending on vaccine or condition			
Meningococcal A, C, W, Y (MenACWY)	1 or 2 doses depending on condition (see cdc.gov for booster recommendations)			
Meningococcal B (MenB)	ages 19–23	2 or 3 doses depending on vaccine or condition (see cdc.gov for booster recommendations)		
Meningococcal B (Hib)	1 or 3 doses depending on indication			
Coronavirus (COVID-19)	3 primary doses plus boosters			

Recommended vaccination for adults who meet age requirement, lack documentation of vaccination, or lack evidence of past infection.

Recommended vaccination for adults with an additional risk factor or another indication.

Recommended vaccination based on shared clinical decision-making.

MASK UP

Mask-wearing exploded into Western consciousness during the COVID-19 pandemic, but in some parts of the world, it's been common courtesy for years. After all, face masks help prevent the spread of ordinary colds and flus, too. Here's how to make sure yours fits properly.

STEP 1: Carry a mask with you when you go out. If it's a cloth mask, it should have multiple layers of tightly woven, breathable fabric. Handle it by the ear loops, cords, or head straps—not by the mask's surface. Avoid masks with valves or vents, since they'll expose other people to your germs.

STEP 2: If you're in a public place (especially indoors), consider wearing a mask, even if there's no global pandemic as you read this.

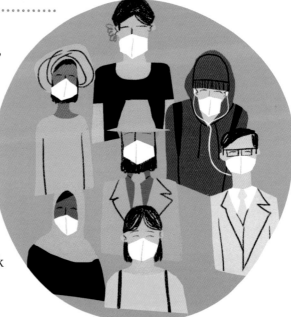

STEP 3: Make sure it completely covers your nose as well as your mouth. Check the edges to make sure there are no gaps between the mask and your face.

☐ If you've covered your nose and mouth with a properly fitting mask in a public place, cover yourself with glory.

DON'T SIT STILL

Much of this book is scientific vindication of the things people told you when you were a kid. Eat your vegetables! Buckle up!

But if your grade school teacher is reading this book, this next tip is going to shatter a core belief. Are you ready, Mrs. Coopersmith? Here we go:

Fidgeting is good for you.

One study that followed 12,778 women for more than a decade found that fidgeting saves lives. Specifically, it breaks the connection between sitting and mortality (page 45). The women who sat for more than seven hours a day had a 30 percent greater risk of mortality...if they didn't fidget much. Self-described fidgeters, on the other hand, seemed to be able to sit for seven hours without increasing their risk of death. Given that this is just one study, it's probably better to avoid prolonged sitting if you can. But if you can't . . . fidget!

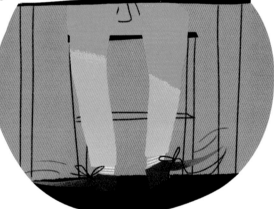

STEP 1: When you sit, get in the habit of jiggling your feet or twirling a pen. Or get a fidget toy and play with it.

☐ If you fidgeted while you sat today, jiggle a crown on your head.

DO AS LITTLE AS POSSIBLE

Throughout this book, I've tried to break down health and fitness into concrete, manageable steps. But life is full of distractions and challenges, and it's easy to get overwhelmed. If that happens to you, remember: Any step forward, no matter how tiny, is better than none.

STEP 1: Identify an area of your health that you'd like to improve. Do you want to eat better? Get more exercise?

STEP 2: If the prospect of change seems overwhelming, identify the smallest possible step you can take. Can you eat a single bite of carrot every day? Attempt a single sit-up?

STEP 3: Take that step. Do it again tomorrow.

STEP 4: When you've done that single step every day for a week, consider adding a second step. You're already eating a bite of carrot. Can you take two?

STEP 5: Keep making incremental improvements at whatever pace feels sustainable to you. If you stick with it, you'll find those ridiculously small tweaks add up to real change.

☐ If you've taken a single step to improve your health and fitness, no matter how small it was, give yourself a massive win.

MOVE HEALTHY

Exercise reduces your risk of cancer, diabetes, heart attack, dementia, and strokes, while extending your life, giving you more energy, and improving your mood. If it were a pill, it would be the blockbuster medical discovery of all time.

Until you can purchase exercise over the counter, here are practical, real-life ways you can integrate it into your daily routine.

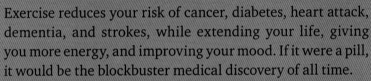

GET AN RX FOR XRCISE

If you don't exercise regularly, or you have any health concerns, you'll definitely want to check with a doctor before you try any of the tips in this section. But even if you're pretty fit already, talking with your doctor before you begin an exercise regimen can have psychological benefits.

STEP 1: Ask your doctor if there's anything you need to know before you start a new exercise regimen.

. . . .

STEP 2: Have your doctor make a note in your records to check in with you next time they see you to find out how your exercise habit is going. Reporting to a health-care professional may make people more likely to stick with a healthy habit.

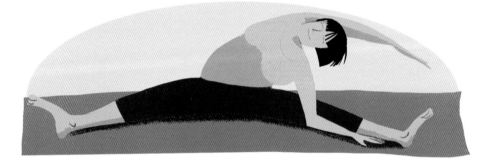

☐ If you've consulted with a doctor about your exercise plans, give yourself the win.

STAND UP FOR YOUR HEALTH

As twenty-first-century primates, we take bodies that evolved to roam vast distances and force them to sit for hours in front of a glowing screen. We're stand-up creatures in a sit-down world.

Not surprisingly, prolonged sitting has all sorts of negative health consequences. It increases the risk of blood clots, weight gain, and insulin resistance, and it may lead to diabetes and dementia.

Fortunately, this is one health problem with a simple cure.

STEP 1: If you're sitting for more than an hour, stand up for at least a minute.

STEP 2: If you can, plan your day to avoid prolonged sitting. Leave your to-do list just out of arm's reach. Take a walk between two video meetings. Some people even get standing desks. If you can't avoid sitting, at least try to fidget (page 41).

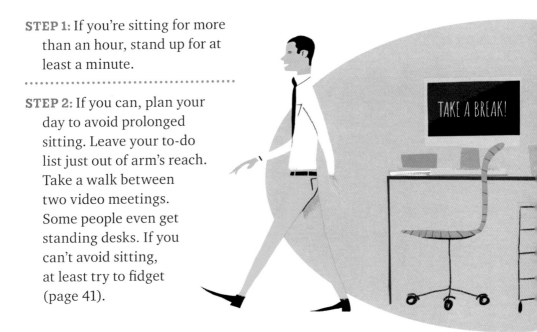

TAKE A BREAK!

☐ If you've interrupted a prolonged session of sitting, give yourself a standing ovation.

SNACK ON EXERCISE

In an ideal world, you'd have hours a day for exercise.

In the real world, you may have a three-minute break between phone calls.

Fortunately, if you can't make a full meal of exercise, you can get real benefit from an exercise snack—any brief, intense bout of physical activity. It can be as short as a few seconds or as long as a few minutes. The more of them you can fit in over your day, the better—but even a single snack two or three times a week can contribute to cardiovascular fitness.

As with all exercise, choose your snack based on your fitness level. You want something that is as intense as you can safely manage, but not overwhelming or injury-risking. Depending on how fit you are, a snack could involve sprinting up the ten-story staircase in your office building or walking slowly down the hallway to look out your window.

It could be picking up your teeny kitten for a quick cuddle or lifting your massive Great Dane ten times over your head. (Just make sure your Great Dane doesn't have a full bladder.)

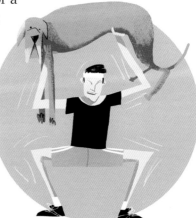

STEP 1: Think about little bursts of exercise you can fit in throughout your day.

STEP 2: When you have a few free minutes, start with a brief gentle warm-up, like walking in place.

STEP 3: Do your exercise snack.

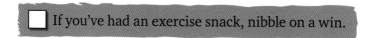

☐ If you've had an exercise snack, nibble on a win.

EXERCISE AT THE RIGHT TIME

No matter when you do it, exercise is good for you. But the time of day you do it may shape exactly what kind of goodness it delivers.

There's some evidence that exercising on an empty stomach before you have breakfast burns more fat, while doing it later in the day helps control blood sugar levels. The latter could be of particular interest to the 122 million Americans who have diabetes or prediabetes.

I don't want to oversell this. The evidence here is intriguing but preliminary. And the best time of day to exercise is always the time you'll actually do it. But if you have options, it may be worth experimenting to find which one works best.

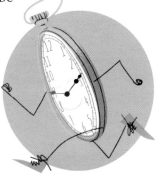

STEP 1: If you have lots of flexibility regarding your exercise schedule, read on. Otherwise, just exercise whenever you can work it in.

STEP 2: If your primary goal is weight loss or maintenance, work out before breakfast.

STEP 3: If your primary goal is blood sugar control, ask your doctor if you should schedule your exercise for the afternoon.

STEP 4: Don't exercise vigorously within an hour of bedtime—it will make it harder to sleep. But a bedtime routine that includes yoga or other gentle stretching can help you drift off more easily.

STEP 5: Don't let your quest for a perfect time interfere with finding a perfectly acceptable time. If your only free moment is after you drop the kids off at 9 AM and before you meet your friend for coffee at 9:15, then go for a jog from 9:01 to 9:14 and don't give it a further thought.

☐ If you've thought about your best time to exercise, take the win.

JOIN THE TEAM

Exercising on your own is good for your body.

Exercising on a team may be good for your soul.

Joining a team has been shown to correlate with improved life satisfaction, thanks to the combination of physical and social activity. Plus, the commitment you make to your peers helps you stick with your exercise goals.

STEP 1: Identify a sport you enjoy (or would like to learn more about).

....

STEP 2: Search on the internet for a team in your area.

....

STEP 3: Show up to a practice and see if you click.

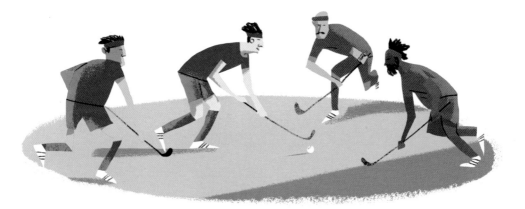

☐ If you've joined a team, shown up for a team practice, or even researched a team in the area, join in the victory celebration.

GET AN EXERCISE BUDDY

I'm pretty good about following my own advice. But I confess: Despite everything I know about the psychological and physical benefits of team sports, I haven't played one since high school, unless you count improv comedy. I'm just not a team sports kind of guy.

Fortunately, I've found a lower-key way to get some of the same social benefits as joining a team: exercising with a friend. Whenever we get the chance, my wife and I take long walks together, and it's one of the highlights of my day.

You might choose your partner depending on what you're going for. Unsurprisingly, the evidence suggests that working out with somebody more fit than you will make you exercise harder—but working out with somebody less fit will make the experience more relaxing.

STEP 1: Find somebody whose company you enjoy, who is interested in doing the same type of exercise as you.

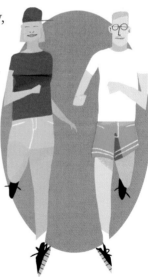

STEP 2: Make an appointment to exercise with them. If it's possible to make it a regular thing—if you can walk a mile together every Tuesday after work—great! If not, schedule it whenever you can.

STEP 3: Exercise together, doing good for your heart and soul.

☐ If you've exercised with a buddy, or made plans to, give both of you a win.

EXERCISE FOR HEALTH, NOT WEIGHT LOSS

Does exercise help you shed fat?

Kind of.

Here's why it *does*:

- In theory, you lose fat when you expend more energy than you take in. An extra 100 calories of exercise should have the same effect as 100 fewer calories of food.
- Exercise can add muscle. Muscles burn more calories even when you're sitting still.
- If you cut calories without exercising, you'll lose muscle as well as fat. Exercise helps signal to your body to keep the muscle it already has.
- Exercise can cause changes in your metabolism that help reduce fat.

And here's why exercise *doesn't* help you lose fat:

- Most people overestimate how much junk food their workout buys them. Let's say you run for thirty minutes and then reward yourself with a glazed doughnut. The run burned off about three hundred calories. The doughnut has about 380 calories. Over the course of the morning, you've gained eighty calories.
- If you burn more calories through activity, your body compensates by burning less energy in its resting state. At least, it compensates partially. If you burn 100 calories exercising, your body burns about twenty-eight fewer calories while resting. Your 100 calories of exercise have earned you only seventy-two calories of weight loss.
- Your body also compensates by making you hungrier, up to a point.

STEP 1: Make the same healthy food decisions whether or not you've recently exercised.

STEP 2: Consider exercise a success if it helps you feel healthier, happier, or more energetic, whether or not your waist size changes.

STEP 3: If you are cutting calories, exercise to make sure you lose weight from fat rather than muscle. Resistance exercises (like weight lifting) seem especially important for maintaining muscle mass.

STEP 4: If you do want to lose weight from exercise, aim for about three thousand calories or three hundred minutes a week. That seems to be the point at which you burn enough calories to overcome your body's compensating mechanisms. Alternatively, regularly include HIIT (page 68), which seems to promote fat-burning.

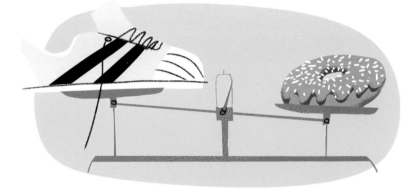

☐ If you've reframed exercise as pro-health rather than anti-fat, you've gained a win.

ACTIVELY EXPERIMENT

If you go for a jog and hate it, it's tempting to conclude that you're destined for the sofa. But physical activity is a breathtakingly broad category. It includes everything from twirling a baton to splitting logs to chasing a dog around the yard. In that vast universe of movement, an option must exist that you will actively enjoy. Find it, and moving your body becomes not an obligation but a highlight of your day.

Things You Can Do to Get Your Body Moving

- Milking cows
- Painting a house
- Swimming
- Carrying a child
- Running up and down the sidelines while coaching a Little League team
- Jumping rope
- Roller-skating
- Snorkeling
- Skiing
- Dancing like an idiot to your favorite song
- Fitness video games
- Martial arts
- Jumping on a trampoline
- Wheelchair basketball
- Lifting weights
- Gardening and yard work
- Hiking
- Yoga

STEP 1: Try two or three forms of physical activity. See the sidebar if you need some inspiration.

STEP 2: Take notes. What did you enjoy? What would you change? Use those to point you toward your next experiment. If you enjoyed the music aspect of a rhythm dancing game but found it lonely, head out for ballroom dance lessons next.

STEP 3: Keep going until you find a form of physical activity you look forward to doing. If you find more than one, even better—varying your routine is good for you (page 56).

☐ If you've found a physical activity you love—or even just taken steps to find it—you've found a win.

PAINT

BE PATIENT WITH YOURSELF

If you rarely or never exercise, the good news is that it's never too late to start. The bad news is that starting may feel miserable.

You might have heard that working out releases feel-good chemicals called endorphins. That's true—but it takes about twenty minutes of vigorous exercise for your body to start producing them. And if you aren't already fit, you may not be able to work out enough to get to that point.

So if you're starting to move your body after a mostly sedentary life, don't give up.

STEP 1: If you aren't in the habit of exercising, and it feels miserable to start, be patient with yourself.

STEP 2: Find any form of exercise you can tolerate. Use the tips in this section to make it as easy and fun as possible. But for now, ignore anything I say about optimal amounts or kinds of exercise. Your near-term goal is just to stick with the habit until your brain begins to reward you for it. (And, of course, to avoid injury—better to go slowly than hurt yourself and have to interrupt your progress.)

STEP 3: Remember that, if you can persist for a few months, working out will seem much less daunting, and the glow you get afterward will feel better and better.

STEP 4: In the meantime, by sticking with it, you are demonstrating more willpower than somebody who is already athletic enough to get the neural rewards. That's right: As far as I'm concerned, you are more impressive than Usain Bolt.

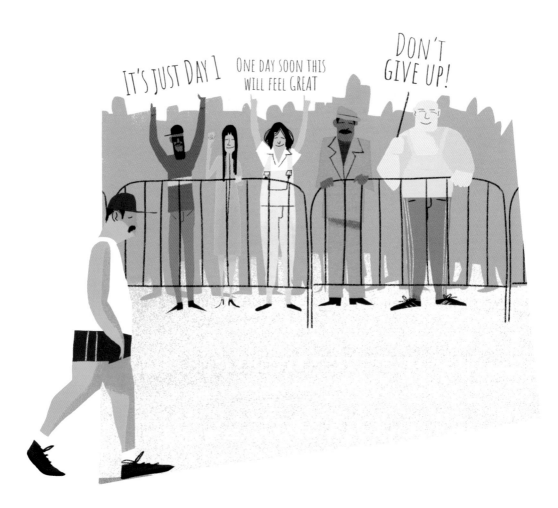

If you've been patient with yourself as you start an exercise habit, you're an Olympic-level winner in my book.

VARY YOUR WORKOUTS

Whatever workout you do, it will become easier with time. That's a good thing—it means you've learned new skills and built new muscles. But to keep challenging yourself, and to make sure you're working out your entire body, introduce some variety into your workout.

When it comes to exercise, variety isn't just the spice of life—it's one of the main ingredients.

STEP 1: If you're doing the same activities over and over again, experiment to find new ones you enjoy (page 52).

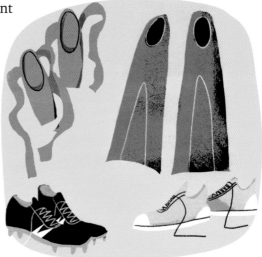

STEP 2: Make sure you're varying the kind of exercise as well. Look for a mix of cardio (page 60), HIIT (page 68), and resistance (page 58) or weight training (page 65).

STEP 3: Even within the same activity, challenge yourself with new varieties. Work on a new karate kata or ballroom dance step. If you're lifting weights, find a different move to target the same muscle—there's evidence that variety promotes muscle growth.

☐ If you've broken up your exercise routine with some variety, your winning streak continues.

DRESS FOR THE WORKOUT YOU WANT

The effort of changing into my workout clothes shouldn't be enough to stop me from working out. Putting on sweatpants takes thirty seconds, and the exercise that ensues could add years to my life.

Alas, I'm a human, and I'm just as dumb as the rest of my species.

If you're smarter than I am, and you never miss a workout, you can skip this tip. But if you're a fellow goofy, inconsistent primate, give it a try.

STEP 1: Before bed, lay out whatever clothes you work out in. Put them someplace impossible to miss. If you exercise when you get home from work, for example, put them in the front hall of your home so you'll see them as soon as you step inside.

STEP 2: When the time comes, put on your workout clothes. Don't think about exercise. You're not committing to anything. Just put those clothes on.

STEP 3: Now that you're dressed for it, you will find it weirdly easier to actually do the exercise.

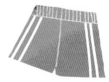

☐ If you've laid out your workout clothes for the next day, put on some victory garb.

ENCOUNTER RESISTANCE

Not everybody can fit an entire weight room into their home. Fortunately, elastic resistance bands are a great way to exhaust your muscles without exhausting your closet—or your budget.

The following exercises are courtesy of the British Heart Foundation.

STEP 1: LATERAL RAISE. Stand with both feet in the middle of the band. Hold one end in each hand. Raise your arms away from your waist until they reach shoulder height. Return to the starting position. Repeat ten times.

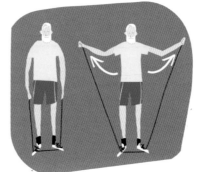

STEP 2: SQUATS. Stand with both feet in the middle of the band. Hold one end in each hand. Slowly bend to a squatting position, as if you were sitting on an invisible chair. Make sure your knees are behind your toes. Return to your starting position. Repeat ten times.

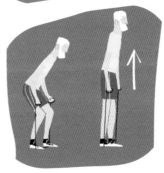

STEP 3: CHEST PRESS. Sitting or standing, put the band behind your back and hold each end. Stretch your arms forward, away from your chest. Return to your starting position. Repeat ten times.

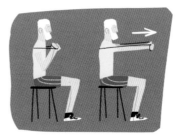

STEP 4: LEG PRESS. Sit with your back straight. Put one foot in the middle of the band, holding both ends with your hands. Bend your knee toward you, then straighten it back out. Repeat ten times.

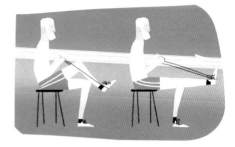

STEP 5: BICEP CURL. Sitting or standing, put your feet in the middle of the band. Hold one end in each hand. Curling your elbow, raise each hand to chest height. Return to starting position. Repeat ten times.

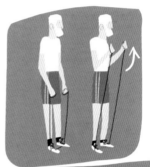

STEP 6: SEATED CALF PRESS. Sit with your back straight. Put one foot in the band and hold both ends with your hands. With your leg extended, point your toes toward the ceiling and then toward the ground. Repeat with each leg ten times.

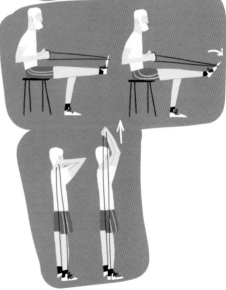

STEP 7: TRICEP PRESS. Stand in the middle of the band with one heel. Holding the band with both hands, stretch it behind your body and pull it above your head. Return to your starting position. Repeat ten times on each side.

☐ If you've done one resistance band workout, it's no stretch to call it a victory.

GET TO 150

Counting your steps (page 62) is a simple way to make sure you get enough exercise. But it's not the only way. If you'd like to try a broader exercise guideline, you might keep two targets in mind.

With just ninety minutes of moderate activity per week, you add three whole years to your life expectancy.

If you can get 150 minutes of moderate activity per week—a mere thirty minutes a day, five days a week—you cut your risk of illness and depression even further. Of course, if you have the time and energy, you can do more— but after about three hundred minutes, the health benefits aren't that big.

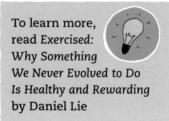

To learn more, read *Exercised: Why Something We Never Evolved to Do Is Healthy and Rewarding* by Daniel Lie

If you don't have 150 minutes a week, or if you just like to sweat, you can move more intensely for a shorter time. Every minute of vigorous activity counts as two minutes of moderate.

If you want to make a precise distinction between vigorous and moderate activity, you can measure your heart rate (page 66). Otherwise, a rough rule of thumb is that moderate activity leaves you with enough breath to carry on a conversation, but not enough to sing. Vigorous activity lets you talk, but it becomes somewhat difficult to carry on a full conversation.

STEP 1: Find an exercise you enjoy, or at least one you can tolerate.

....

STEP 2: Get thirty minutes of moderate activity today, or fifteen minutes of vigorous activity.

....

STEP 3: If you're having fun and you feel good, keep going.

....

STEP 4: Repeat at least five times a week.

- Brisk walking
- Active cleaning like mopping or vacuuming
- Pushing an electric lawn mower
- Biking at around ten mph
- Line dancing
- Boxing with a punching bag

- Hiking
- Jogging
- Shoveling snow
- Playing soccer
- Biking around fifteen mph
- Energetic square dancing
- Boxing in the ring

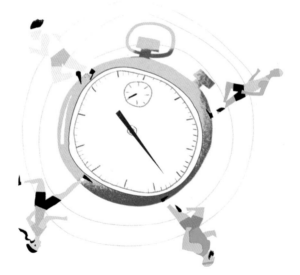

☐ If you got thirty minutes of moderate activity or fifteen minutes of vigorous activity today, give your back-patting arm a workout.

TAKE THE STEPS

How many steps a day do you really need?

The well-known recommendation of ten thousand steps a day was invented in 1965 by a Japanese company that was trying to sell pedometers.

In 2019, a more rigorous study of nearly seventeen thousand women found that people who took 4,400 steps per day lived longer than people who took 2,700. The more steps you took, the better—up until 7,500 steps a day. Going beyond 7,500 steps didn't seem to affect lifespan either way.

STEP 1: Get something to measure your steps. It doesn't have to be fancy—you can get a decent pedometer that clips to your belt for under fifteen bucks. If you own a smartphone, it may have this function built in or available as an inexpensive app.

STEP 2: Aim for at least 4,400 steps a day. If you've got that under control, set your sights on 7,500.

☐ If you've tracked your step count and worked on increasing it, take the step of acknowledging your win.

FIGHT FOR THE WORST PARKING SPACE

Even if you can't work a full 4,400 steps into your busy day, you can always add more steps than you're used to—and every one will be a step in the right direction.

STEP 1: When you drive somewhere, park your car in the farthest space from the entrance. If there's no lot and you're parking on the street, park at least two blocks away.

STEP 2: If your destination is less than a mile away, skip the car entirely and just walk or bike there. That's not just good for your heart—it's good for the environment and your wallet, since short car trips are the most fuel-inefficient.

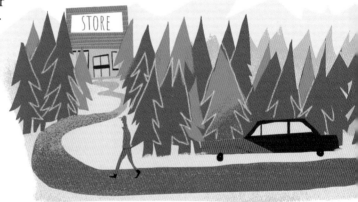

STEP 3: Any time you take an elevator, get off one floor early and take the stairs.

☐ If you added even one extra minute of walking to your daily routine, stroll over to the victory circle.

DON'T STRETCH IT

For years, coaches insisted that you stretch before a workout to prevent injury. It turns out they had it backward, at least in some sports.

In sports that involve sprinting, stretching before you begin may have some benefit. But in endurance sports, like long-distance running, stretching right before a workout makes your performance worse, and it may increase your risk of injury.

The evidence is more mixed on stretching *after* a workout, but it seems less likely to cause an injury, and it may help reduce soreness.

To be clear, I'm talking about *static stretching*, where you stretch a muscle until it feels tight and then hold the pose. There may be value to *dynamic stretching* (sometimes just called *warming up*), where you gently move your muscles through a comfortable range of motion.

STEP 1: If you're about to go for a long-distance run, or any other sport where you risk overusing a muscle or joint, don't stretch beforehand. Instead, warm up with a brisk walk or a light jog.

STEP 2: If you stretch regularly as part of your exercise routine—if you do yoga, for example—don't do it right before a session of endurance exercise. Wait at least ten minutes.

STEP 3: After your workout, cool down to prevent soreness (page 78). If you want, you can

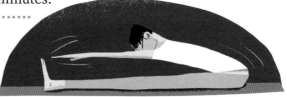

stretch afterward. Pay attention to your own body, and note whether stretching makes you more or less achy the next day.

☐ If you took a thoughtful, informed approach to stretching, it's no stretch to call it a win.

MUSCLE UP

When we talk about exercise, we often emphasize its benefits for the heart and lungs. Yes, the cardiovascular system is pretty darn important. But your heart isn't the only muscle the matters.

Exercises that work your other muscles make you physically stronger, and many people like the aesthetic effect as well. Oh, and as a teeny bonus, they may strengthen your bones, improve your brain function, reduce your blood pressure, lower your risk of falling, and ease back pain and arthritis.

STEP 1: Find a muscle-building activity that you enjoy—or at least can tolerate. The possibilities don't just end with lifting weights. You can also work out with resistance bands (page 58) or your own body weight (page 70).

STEP 2: Work your legs, hips, back, chest, abdomen, shoulders, and arms, at least twice a week.

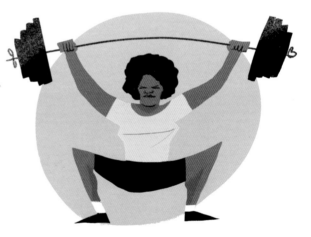

STEP 3: Gradually increase the amount of weight you're working with (or the resistance of the bands).

☐ If you did muscle-building exercises today (or you've done it twice this week), you're a heavyweight champion.

FIGURE OUT YOUR MAX HEART RATE

The more intense the exercise, the faster your heart beats . . . up to a point. Eventually, your heart hits a hard upper limit, called your *maximum heart rate* or *HRMax*. If you know what that limit is, you can target your workouts more precisely.

High-intensity interval training (page 68) aims to get your heart rate to 80 percent or more of the maximum.

Active recovery (page 78) aims to keep your heart at 50 percent to 60 percent of its maximum.

Don't Worry

Calculating your max heart rate is not a requirement for leading a healthy life! This tip is purely for data-hungry self-measurement junkies.

What Different Heart Rates Do for You

How much exercise you do per week (page 60) depends on whether it's moderate or vigorous activity.

- "Moderate activity" is a workout that gets your heart rate to 64 percent to 76 percent of its maximum.

- "Vigorous activity" is a workout that gets your heart rate to between 77 percent and 94 percent of its maximum.

STEP 1: Multiply your age by 0.64. Subtract that number from 211. The number you get is a pretty good estimate of maximum heart rate.

$$50 \times .64 = 32$$
$$211 - 32 = 179$$

I'm fifty, so my maximum heart rate is 179 beats per minute.

STEP 2: If you've got a fitness tracker with a built-in heart monitor, you can get an even more accurate and personalized measure. Pick an aerobic exercise like jogging, and warm up to the point where you're sweating.

STEP 3: Now speed up, pushing yourself hard enough that you can't talk. Keep it up for four minutes, then walk briskly for three minutes to rest.

STEP 4: Do another round, with another intense four minutes followed by a three-minute rest.

STEP 5: Start a third round, but two minutes, speed up as fast as you can and run until you're too exhausted to continue. Your HRMax is the fastest rate your heart reached.

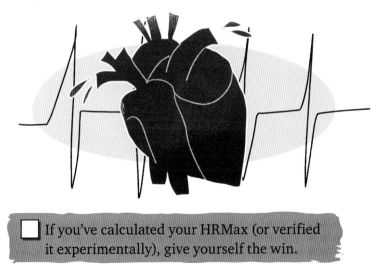

☐ If you've calculated your HRMax (or verified it experimentally), give yourself the win.

TAKE A HIIT

If you want maximum physical benefit in minimum time, the good news is: There's a workout that will strengthen your cardiovascular system and help you lose fat in less than thirty minutes, two or three times a week.

The bad news: It's going to be a very challenging thirty minutes.

High-intensity interval training, or *HIIT*, involves intervals of pushing yourself so hard you can't talk in complete sentences, interspersed with "rests" like jogging or brisk walking. Most people shouldn't do it more than two or three times a week. (Serious athletes may be able to handle it more often, but that's a question to discuss with a professional trainer.)

There are many kinds of HIIT, and it's not clear if any one of them is better than any other. I've chosen this one because it's one of the most commonly studied.

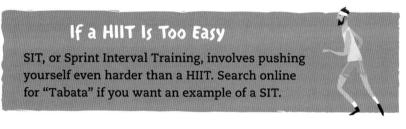

If a HIIT Is Too Easy

SIT, or Sprint Interval Training, involves pushing yourself even harder than a HIIT. Search online for "Tabata" if you want an example of a SIT.

STEP 1: High-intensity interval training is . . . well, highly intense. If you're not already exercising regularly, or if you have any medical condition, check with your doctor before starting it.

STEP 2: Walk briskly or jog for ten minutes to warm up. Or, if you want to go easier on your knees, pedal a stationary bike at an easy pace.

STEP 3: Run or pedal your stationary bike for four minutes. Aim for a pace where, after a minute or two, you're breathing heavily and can't speak in complete sentences. Aim for 85 percent to 95 percent of HRMax if you know it (page 66). Don't go so hard that you can't finish the four-minute set.

STEP 4: Take an active break. Walk briskly, jog, or pedal gently for three minutes. (If you know your HRMax, aim for 60 percent of it.) The idea is to slow down enough to rest, while keeping your blood pumping just enough to clear soreness-causing lactic acid from your muscles.

STEP 5: Do three more intense exercise/active recovery cycles for a total of four.

STEP 6: End with five more minutes of brisk walking or moderate pedaling to cool down.

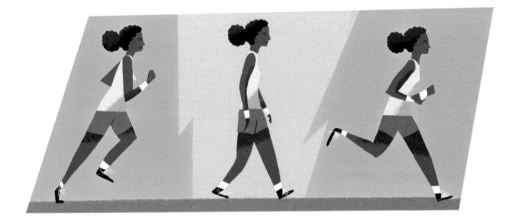

☐ If you've done a HIIT session, take an intense win.

SEVEN MINUTES TO FITNESS

On page 68, we talked about a HIIT routine involving running. But some studies suggest that all-out bursts of body-weight exercises (like push-ups or squats) can also whip your cardiovascular system into shape.

With no equipment beyond a chair, you can blitz a wide variety of muscle groups. This particular routine was developed by Chris Jordan, an exercise physiologist who has advised the British army and the US Air Force. But there's nothing magical about it. Feel free to substitute a different workout for the same body part. And if it's too hard for you, don't risk injury! Check out the more gentle version on page 72.

If you search "J&J Official 7-minute workout" in the Android or iPhone app store, you can find Jordan's free app, which will let you tailor the workout to your personal fitness level.

STEP 1: Look over the entire workout. If there's any exercise you're not familiar with, look it up on the video site of your choice. You'll be pushing yourself hard, and to avoid injury, you'll want to make sure you've got good form.

STEP 2: Do thirty seconds of jumping jacks. On an intensity scale of one to ten, aim for an effort level of about eight. In other words, push yourself nearly (but not quite) as hard as you can.

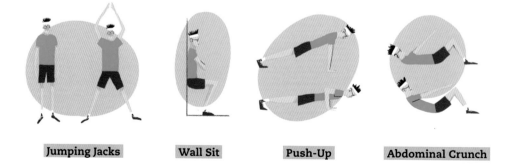

Jumping Jacks   Wall Sit   Push-Up   Abdominal Crunch

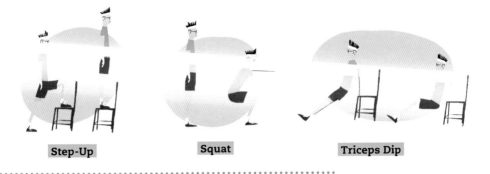

Step-Up   **Squat**   **Triceps Dip**

STEP 3: Rest for ten seconds.

STEP 4: Do thirty seconds of the next exercise in the workout.

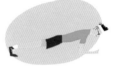

Plank

STEP 5: Rest for ten seconds.

STEP 6: Keep alternating exercise and rest until you've completed the full workout.

STEP 7: Believe it or not, if you do the seven-minute workout often enough, you'll build up enough strength to have energy left at the end. When you get to that stage, you can do the whole thing twice, for an even more vigorous fourteen-minute workout.

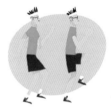

High Knees

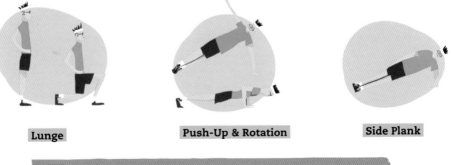

Lunge   **Push-Up & Rotation**   **Side Plank**

☐ If you've done the seven-minute workout, spend a few extra seconds on acknowledging your win.

SEVEN MORE GENTLE MINUTES TO FITNESS

In 2013, the *New York Times* published Chris Jordan's Seven-Minute Workout (page 70). It helped a lot of people (including me) fit an intense body-weight workout into their busy lives.

But it wasn't for everybody. Not everybody's knees are up to jumping jacks, nor can everybody comfortably get down on the floor for a push-up and then stand back up. And so, in 2021, the *Times* and Jordan collaborated on a more gentle version of the Seven-Minute Workout.

If you search for "Chris Jordan Standing 7 Minute Workout," you can find a video of Mr. Jordan demonstrating it himself, but for now, here's a summary.

STEP 1: Do the first exercise on the circuit for thirty seconds.

....

STEP 2: Rest for five seconds, then move on to the next one. For any exercise you can't quite manage, feel free to do a slower version, or one with a smaller range of motion.

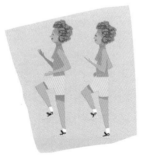

Marching in place

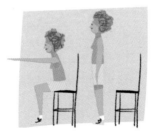

Chair-assist squat

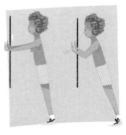

Wall push-up (round 1)

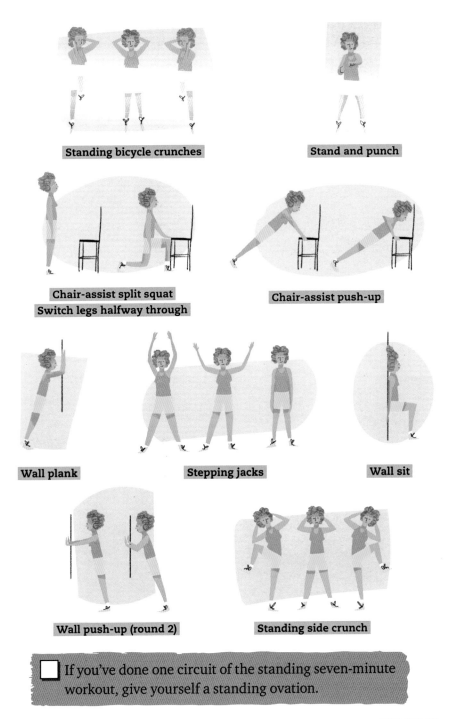

Standing bicycle crunches

Stand and punch

Chair-assist split squat
Switch legs halfway through

Chair-assist push-up

Wall plank

Stepping jacks

Wall sit

Wall push-up (round 2)

Standing side crunch

☐ If you've done one circuit of the standing seven-minute workout, give yourself a standing ovation.

FOUR FRANTIC SECONDS TO FITNESS

As I discussed earlier (page 45), extended sitting is surprisingly bad for your health. Fortunately, even if you're not a natural fidgeter (page 41), there's still hope.

According to a small but intriguing study, four-second sprints of frantic, all-out exercise may help prevent some of the metabolic dangers of extended sitting.

I want to be clear: This is not a magic recipe for total fitness. Nobody ever made it to the Olympics through four-second bursts of jumping jacks. But if you're stuck at your desk all day, it's worth getting your blood pumping in whatever tiny sprints you can manage.

STEP 1: On days when you have to sit for hours and don't have time for extensive exercise, set a timer to go off once an hour.

STEP 2: When the timer goes off, exercise all out for four seconds. You might do jumping jacks or sprint in place or pedal frantically on a stationary bike.

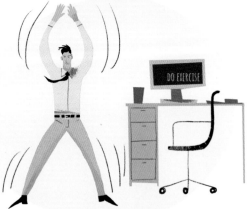

STEP 3: Give yourself forty-five seconds of rest.

STEP 4: Repeat the four-second exercise/forty-five-second rest pattern four more times for a total of five.

☐ If you've broken up an hour of sitting as described, frantically give yourself the win.

TUNE UP YOUR FORM

When I was on my high school swim team, I never bothered to learn proper technique. As a fast-healing teenager, I got away with it. When I returned to swimming in my forties, my poor form finally caught up with me. My back seized up completely. As soon as I could walk upright again, I booked a single session with an expert in swim technique. He filmed me swimming, pointed out exactly what I was doing wrong, and sent me off.

Whether you swim, bowl, or dance the cha-cha, a brief but intense focus on proper form can prevent a lifetime of injuries.

STEP 1: Identify a form of exercise you perform regularly (or would like to).

STEP 2: Find an instructor who specializes in proper form. If there's a local association focused on your activity, it might be able to point you in the right direction. Or contact a shop that sells relevant equipment or try a web search.

COACH

STEP 3: Book a session with the instructor. Emphasize that you are interested in making this activity sustainable and injury-free in the long term.

STEP 4: Show up for the session and learn how to do it right.

☐ If you've booked or attended a session with an expert in form, give yourself a smooth, flowing pat on the back.

TWEAK YOUR BODY WEIGHT

When you start lifting barbells, you can adjust the weight to give yourself precisely the right amount of challenge. You can't do that with body-weight exercises, unless you've got some detachable limbs. Fortunately, there *are* things you can do to match body-weight exercises to your current fitness level.

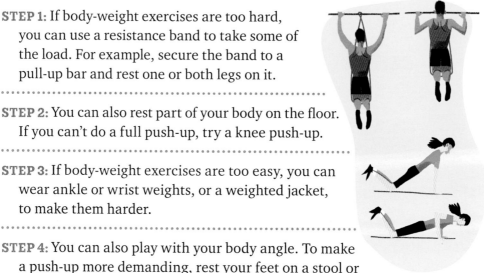

STEP 1: If body-weight exercises are too hard, you can use a resistance band to take some of the load. For example, secure the band to a pull-up bar and rest one or both legs on it.

STEP 2: You can also rest part of your body on the floor. If you can't do a full push-up, try a knee push-up.

STEP 3: If body-weight exercises are too easy, you can wear ankle or wrist weights, or a weighted jacket, to make them harder.

STEP 4: You can also play with your body angle. To make a push-up more demanding, rest your feet on a stool or chair. (Make sure you're stable!)

STEP 5: Don't forget: You can also make body-weight exercises more challenging just by doing more reps of the same move. Sometimes, that's all you need.

STEP 6: Before trying a new version of an exercise, it's always good to find videos of well-trained athletes doing the move you want to do. Proper form reduces your risk of injury.

☐ If you've modified a body-weight exercise to give yourself a greater or lesser challenge, give yourself the win.

EXERCISE LESS

Exercise is one of the most effective medicines there is—but like all medicines, it's possible to overdose.

When you exercise, you deliberately make little tears to the muscles you use (including your heart). When you rest, your body responds to that damage by building back the muscle a little stronger than before. But if you do too much exercise and not enough resting, your body never gets the chance to repair the damage. You get weaker, rather than stronger.

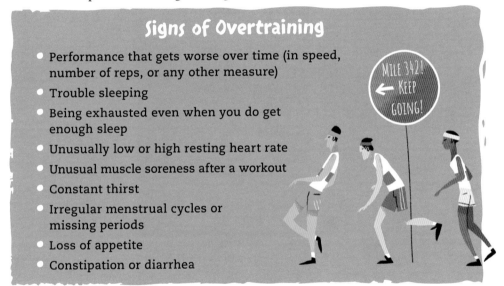

Signs of Overtraining

- Performance that gets worse over time (in speed, number of reps, or any other measure)
- Trouble sleeping
- Being exhausted even when you do get enough sleep
- Unusually low or high resting heart rate
- Unusual muscle soreness after a workout
- Constant thirst
- Irregular menstrual cycles or missing periods
- Loss of appetite
- Constipation or diarrhea

MILE 342! ← KEEP GOING!

STEP 1: If you think you're suffering from overtraining, speak to a doctor or coach.

STEP 2: They may have you cut your training back by 50 percent or more. Listen to the expert, and be patient as you slowly return to a healthy level of exercise.

☐ If you've taken action after spotting warning signs of overtraining, or even just kept an eye out for them, take a nice, relaxing, gentle win.

COOL IT, KID

As you work your muscles intensely, they build up lactic acid. Afterward, you feel sore until the lactic acid is flushed from your body. With active recovery (keeping your heart rate up for a little while after a workout) you can get rid of that soreness faster.

STEP 1: After you finish a workout, keep moving! You don't have to exercise the same muscles; if you've just finished a rock-climbing workout, for example, you can cool down with a walk.

STEP 2: Aim to keep your pulse at about 60 percent of your maximum heart rate rate, if you know it (page 66). If not, just slow down until you could carry on a conversation without running out of breath. (NOTE: Do not carry on a conversation if you are swimming, unless you are a mermaid.)

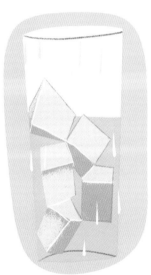

STEP 3: Cool down for ten to thirty minutes. The more intense the workout, the longer you should plan on cooling down. But even if you have to cut your cooldown short, it will still be better than no cooldown at all.

☐ If you've ended a workout with a cooldown, you're hot stuff.

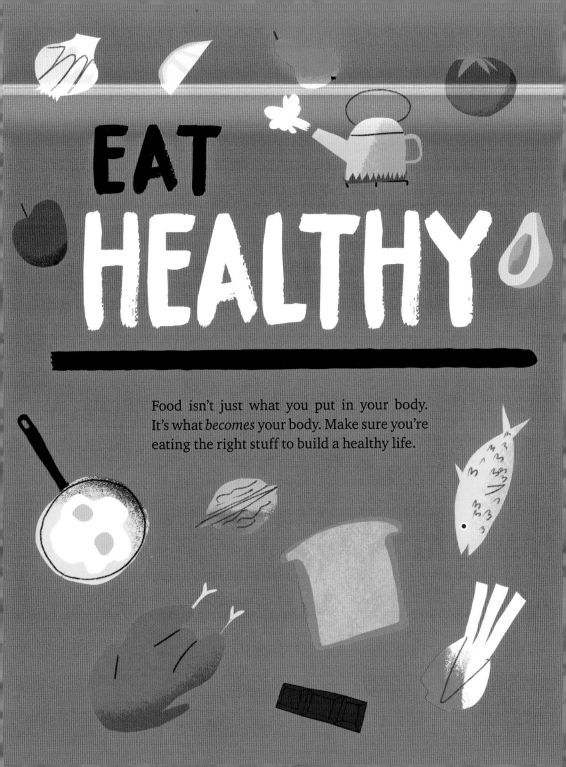

EAT
HEALTHY

Food isn't just what you put in your body. It's what *becomes* your body. Make sure you're eating the right stuff to build a healthy life.

AVOID THE PROCESS

In the language of food science, an apple is an *unprocessed food*.

If you make it into a homemade apple pie, you have a *low-processed food*.

If you add propylene glycol, monostearate, and sodium stearoyl lactylate to your recipe and churn out an ocean of identical plastic-wrapped pies, you now have an *ultra-processed food*.

As that initially healthy apple moved farther and farther from its original state, it lost valuable nutrients and gained large amounts of fat and sugar. The resulting snack cakes have been scientifically engineered to be cheap, shelf-stable, and addictive, with little concern for the health consequences.

Ultra-processed food makes up between 25 percent and 50 percent of the Western diet. And it may be killing us. Ultra-processed food has been linked to obesity, cancer risk, hypertension, and a host of other ailments.

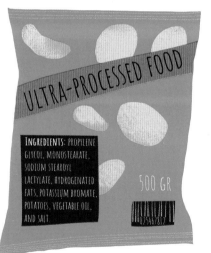

STEP 1: Before you buy a food product, look at the ingredient list. If it contains mysterious-sounding ingredients that you can't buy separately, it is probably ultra-processed food.

STEP 2: Put the ultra-processed food back on the shelf.

STEP 3: Find an alternative that is not ultra-processed. If you want something crunchy and salty, can you buy some nuts? If you want a sweet, prepackaged convenience food, can you get prewashed fruit?

☐ If you've replaced one ultra-processed food with a healthier alternative, give yourself the win.

QUIT YOUR DIET

Every year seems to bring a new bestselling weight-loss diet. The South Beach Diet! The Paleo Diet! The Eat Copies of *Be Healthier Now* Diet! (I'm hoping that last one catches on.)

Many of these diets do work in the short term. If you limit what kind of food you eat, you're likely to consume fewer calories. Unfortunately, when you lose a lot of weight quickly, you often lose muscle mass along with fat. And in the long term, weight-loss diets are hard to sustain—so hard that, as the years go by, the most frequent dieters actually gain the most weight.

Endlessly churning through diet books might be healthy for the publishing industry. But you? You're better off making simple, positive changes to your eating habits.

STEP 1: Before you make any changes to your diet, consider whether you have an unhealthy relationship with food (page 2).

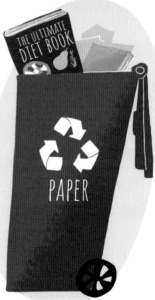

STEP 2: Forget about whatever trendy weight-loss diet your cousin-in-law's barber lost fifty pounds with.

STEP 3: Instead of making huge changes to your eating habits, look for small, positive, and sustainable changes. (This section is full of them!)

☐ If you've shifted your food focus from a crash diet to healthy, sustainable steps, give yourself the win.

COOK FOR YOURSELF

Is that side of cooked carrots at your favorite restaurant delicious because of the chef's skill? Or because they put an entire stick of butter in every serving?

By making your own food, you can exercise control over what you put in your own body.

Home cooking doesn't have to be fancy. A tuna sandwich counts just as much as a lobster bisque. And if you don't consider yourself a good cook, don't worry. Your long-term goal is to find delicious and healthy recipes (page 111). But take it one step at a time. The first step to preparing great meals is just to prepare *something*.

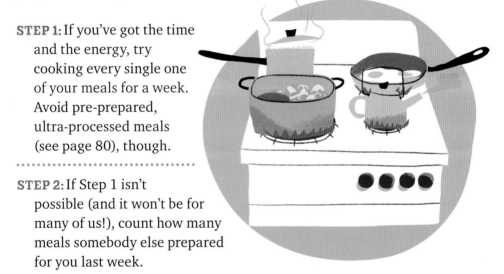

STEP 1: If you've got the time and the energy, try cooking every single one of your meals for a week. Avoid pre-prepared, ultra-processed meals (see page 80), though.

STEP 2: If Step 1 isn't possible (and it won't be for many of us!), count how many meals somebody else prepared for you last week.

STEP 3: Try to eat at least one more home-cooked meal this week.

☐ If you've cooked one more meal for yourself this week, cook up a victory celebration.

PLAN AHEAD

We've all been there. It's the end of a long day, and you suddenly realize you have no idea what you're making for dinner. So you grab whatever's in the fridge, or buy an ultra-processed convenience meal, or order takeout. None of these are recipes for a healthy meal.

It's not surprising, therefore, that a study of more than forty thousand people found that meal planning was associated with healthier and more varied meals, and lower rates of obesity.

STEP 1: Sit down with your calendar and look at the week ahead. What meals will you eat at home?

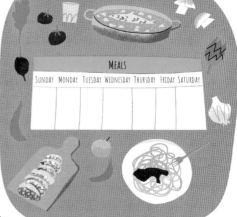

STEP 2: Plan out what you'll make for each one. It doesn't have to be anything fancy. Be realistic about what you can accomplish at the end of a long workday.

STEP 3: Make a shopping plan. When will you buy the ingredients you'll need?

STEP 4: While you're planning, consider doing some advance prep as well. Can you measure the dry ingredients for those whole wheat muffins on Sunday afternoon? That way, you just have to add an egg and some water when you get home from work on Tuesday.

STEP 5: When the day comes, put your plan into action.

☐ If you've planned a future meal, or executed a meal plan you made in the past, give yourself a win.

SPICE UP YOUR LIFE

If you think healthy diets are bland, you've got it backward.

Herbs and spices are good for you. Ginger, cardamom, cinnamon, turmeric, allspice, clove, basil, coriander, fenugreek, caraway, black pepper, dill, rosemary, saffron, and garlic have all been studied for their health benefits. Some may reduce your risk of Alzheimer's and cancer. Some may keep your gut bacteria healthy (page 133). Some may lower inflammation. Many of them are sources of healthy antioxidants and polyphenols.

And if you're having trouble cutting back on salt, consider adding chili. There's evidence that eating spicy foods alters the way you perceive flavor, reducing your desire for salt. As a bonus, eating fresh chili has been linked to a lower risk of cancer, heart disease, and diabetes.

To be clear, spices aren't magic. If you have a deep-fried BLT on a sliced doughnut, adding basil isn't going to make it a healthy meal. And while one spice or another may grab the headlines on any given day, there's no one magic spice; for optimum flavor and nutrition, try a wide variety.

It may be good for your body. It's definitely good for your taste buds.

STEP 1: Seek out recipes that involve a variety of herbs and spices.

STEP 2: Enjoy them.

☐ If you've added more herbs and spices to your diet, enjoy a tasty victory.

There's a nearly infinite variety of herb/food combinations you might enjoy. Consider these few examples a jumping-off point for your own herbal adventures.

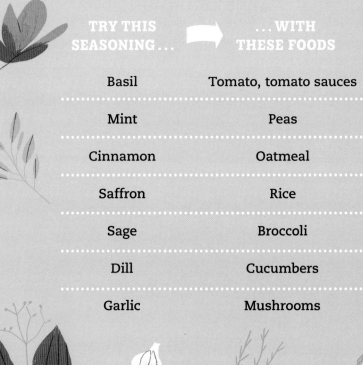

TRY THIS SEASONING...	...WITH THESE FOODS
Basil	Tomato, tomato sauces
Mint	Peas
Cinnamon	Oatmeal
Saffron	Rice
Sage	Broccoli
Dill	Cucumbers
Garlic	Mushrooms

DON'T BE DENSE

Besides the nonfiction Be Better Now series, I've written some children's novels involving a giant pig who lives in a magical river beneath London. Yet as vivid as my imagination is, I can't compare to the greatest fiction writers of our age: the people who come up with serving sizes.

A single serving of Double Stuf Oreos is only 140 calories—because a single serving of Double Stuf Oreos is *two cookies*. If you find somebody who eats two Oreos and stops, let me know. I'd love to introduce them to my giant, magical pig.

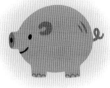

So forget about serving size. Instead, compare foods based on equal weights. One hundred grams of Double Stuf Oreos have 482 calories. By contrast, 100 grams of grapes have about sixty calories. In scientific terms, the Oreos have higher caloric density. More simply, if I want something sweet while keeping my daily calories steady, I can fill my stomach with a lot more grapes than Oreos.

Why Grams?

Grab a couple of food packages, and check out the serving sizes. On one, it might say "two cookies (29 grams)." Another might say "one tablespoon (2 ml)," while a third is "one half cup (50 grams)."

Notice a pattern? Manufacturers are free to label serving sizes in whatever weird unit they want...but by law, they have to convert it to grams or milliliters.

That's why I suggest paying attention to calories per 100 grams. If you're not used to thinking in metric, it might seem a little weird—but it's much easier than trying to compare cookies versus tablespoons versus cups. You'll get the hang of it faster than you think!

STEP 1: If you're trying to decide between two foods, choose the one with the fewest calories per 100 grams. (If it's labeled in milliliters, just treat milliliters like grams. That's not completely precise, but it's good enough for this exercise.)

STEP 2: If the label only tells you how many calories there are in a "serving size," you may have to do a little math. Figure out how many times the serving size goes into 100. Then multiply that by the number of calories. If math isn't your forte, a rough estimate is fine.

A 41-gram serving of Hershey's Kisses has 200 calories.

41 grams goes into 100 about two-and-a-half times.

100 grams has about 500 calories.

STEP 3: Don't view this as a diet (page 81) or a quick weight-loss fix. There's no magic number above which you must never go. The idea is to gradually educate yourself on the caloric density of different foods and to eat more often on the less dense end of the spectrum.

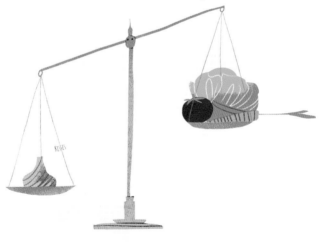

☐ If you've minded the caloric density of your food, consider it a victory-dense meal.

GET A MEAT THERMOMETER

Undercooked meat can be a hotbed of dangerous bacteria. With a quick-reading meat thermometer, you can cook that chicken breast to a temperature that kills germs without killing taste or texture. I promise you: This is one area where health and deliciousness go hand in hand.

That said, if you're a carnivore, a healthy diet may involve shifting your tastes a bit. Red meat consumption (and especially the consumption of processed red meat) is associated with a number of health risks.

STEP 1: Consider replacing beef and pork with chicken and fish. In particular, avoid processed and ultra-processed red meat (page 80 [Avoid the Process]).

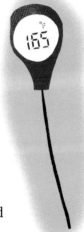

STEP 2: Get a quick-reading, food-safe thermometer. Check your meat in several places, and make sure that the coolest spot has reached the FDA-safe temperature for food.

STEP 3: Some meat thermometers can go inside the oven and alert you when your meat reaches doneness. This lets you take it out the instant it's safe for a moister and tastier result.

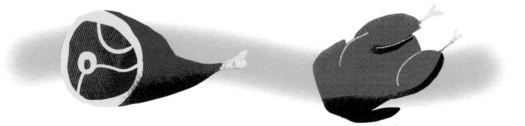

According to the FDA, here are the minimum safe internal temperatures for various meats.

Beef, pork, veal & lamb steaks, chops, roasts	➡	145°F (62.8°C) and allow to rest for at least 3 minutes
Ground meats	➡	160°F (71.1°C)
Ham, fresh or smoked (uncooked)	➡	145°F (62.8°C) and allow to rest for at least 3 minutes
Fully cooked ham (to reheat)	➡	Reheat cooked hams packaged in USDA-inspected plants to 140°F (60°C) and all others to 165°F (73.9°C).
All poultry (breasts, whole bird, ground poultry, giblets, etc.)	➡	165°F (73.9°C)
Fish & shellfish	➡	145°F (62.8°C)
Leftovers & casseroles	➡	165°F (73.9°C)

☐ If you've taken steps to enjoy meat more safely, feast on a win.

ACT FISHY

"Fish, fish—they're good for your heart.
The more you eat, the more you're smart."

I'm sure all of us remember learning that rhyme on the playground. And by "all of us," I mean "me." And by "remember learning that rhyme on the playground," I mean, "making it up a few minutes ago."

If for some reason my poetic genius isn't enough to convince you, allow me to cite a wide variety of peer-reviewed studies. Seafood contains a wealth of nutrients and is lower in unhealthy fats than beef or pork. Eating seafood may reduce your risk of heart disease, cancer, and even depression.

For babies and children, the calculation is a little more complex. The good news: Seafood can be an excellent source of omega-3 fatty acids and other important nutrients for growing young brains. The bad news: Seafood can be a source of mercury and other forms of pollution. The best news: Science can tell us which fish are high in nutrients and low in pollution.

As I write this, the FDA recommends that anybody who is pregnant or breastfeeding have two or three weekly servings from their "best choices" list, or one weekly serving from the "good choices list." (A serving is four ounces.) Recommended amounts for children depend on their age. If you're pregnant, breastfeeding, or otherwise responsible for a small but growing brain, check the FDA website or ask your doctor for the latest recommendations.

Best Choices

Anchovy • Atlantic croaker • Atlantic mackerel • Black sea bass
Butterfish • Catfish • Clam • Cod • Crab • Crawfish • Flounder
Haddock • Hake • Herring • Lobster (American and spiny)
Mullet • Oyster • Pacific chub mackerel • Perch • Pickerel
Plaice • Pollock • Salmon • Sardine • Scallop • Shad • Shrimp
Skate • Smelt • Sole • Squid • Tilapia • Freshwater trout
Canned light tuna (including skipjack) • Whitefish • Whiting

Bluefish Buffalo fish Chilean carp Sea bass/Patagonian toothfish
Grouper Halibut Mahi mahi/dolphinfish Monkfish Rockfish Sablefish
Sheepshead • Snapper • Spanish mackeral • Striped bass (ocean)
Tilefish (from the Atlantic Ocean) • Albacore tuna/White tuna
Yellowfin tuna • Weakfish/seatrout • White croaker/Pacific croaker

Avoid This Seafood. It's High in Mercury.

King mackerel • Marlin • Shark • Swordfish • Orange roughy
Tilefish (from the Gulf of Mexico) • Bigeye tuna

STEP 1: Grown-ups who aren't pregnant or nursing (and don't plan on becoming pregnant) should eat at least one portion of seafood a week. If you can eat more, that's even better.

STEP 2: Aim for baked, grilled, broiled, or steamed. Frying adds unhealthy fat.

STEP 3: If you're a vegetarian, consider adding seaweed to your diet. It's high in fiber and has nutrients that may lower bad cholesterol levels and reduce your risk of cardiovascular disease. Some varieties are good sources of healthy omega-3 fatty acids.

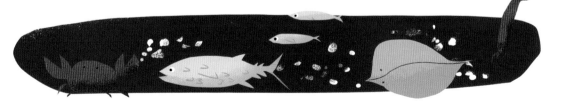

☐ If you've had one serving of seafood today, swim a victory lap.

FILL UP ON FIBER

And the award for Least Glamorous Thing That Is Essential to Your Health goes to . . . fiber! Congratulations, fiber! How'd you do it?

"It's simple, Jacob. I'm vital to blood sugar control and intestinal health. But you know what the most obvious sign is that you're getting enough of me? Regular poops. Can't get less glamorous than that! It's no wonder that most Americans only get half as much fiber as they need!"

Uh . . . Okay. Well, congratulations, fiber!

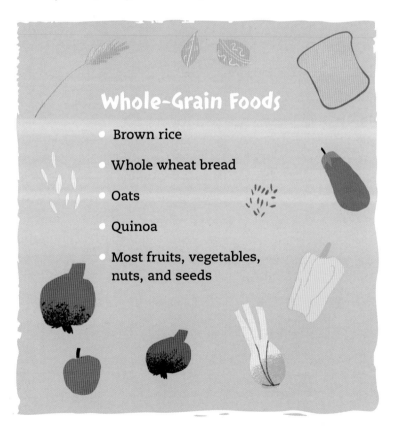

Whole-Grain Foods

- Brown rice
- Whole wheat bread
- Oats
- Quinoa
- Most fruits, vegetables, nuts, and seeds

STEP 1: If you eat processed, low-fiber carbohydrates (like white bread, white rice, or regular pasta), look for whole-grain substitutes.

STEP 2: Be patient with yourself as you make the transition. After making white rice just the way you like it for years, it may take time to find a whole-grain rice you like. If you don't like the first substitute you find, keep experimenting (page 111).

STEP 3: Be creative in your substitutions. You don't have to swap white rice for brown rice. You could swap it for quinoa. You can even put your stir-fry on whole wheat bread. Go wild! The stir-fry police are powerless to stop you!

STEP 4: Increase your fiber intake gradually so your body can get used to the new normal. If you find yourself getting gassy or bloated, or having other unpleasant dietary symptoms, it doesn't mean your system will never handle fiber. It just means you're changing your intake too quickly.

STEP 5: Assuming your gut is behaving, don't stop with substitutions—look for additions as well. How about a handful of raspberries for a midafternoon snack?

STEP 6: Make sure you're drinking enough water (page 104) to help the fiber move through your system.

☐ If you've swapped one low-fiber food for a high-fiber alternative, fill up on victory.

EAT OUT SAFELY

After you've eaten at a restaurant, leftovers are a lovely way to extend the happy experience. Food poisoning? Not so much.

STEP 1: Before you eat out, spend a minute or two to make sure the restaurant's food-safety record is up to snuff. In some areas, restaurants are required to post the results of their latest health inspection on the front door. In others, you may need to search them out on your local department of health website.

STEP 2: Refrigerate leftovers within two hours. That's two hours after it was cooked—not two hours after you leave the restaurant.

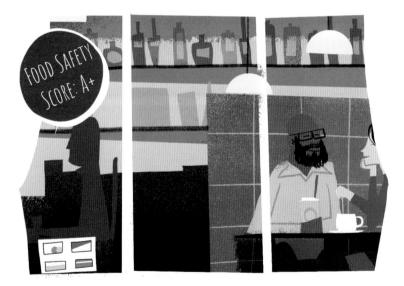

☐ If you've made sure your restaurant meal is as safe as it is delicious, take home a win.

PUT DOWN THE BOTTLE

Bottled water and tap water both rank among the great triumphs of our age.

It's just that tap water is a public health triumph, while bottled water is a marketing triumph.

After all, bottled water exposes you to a vastly greater quantity of potentially harmful microplastics than tap water. Bottled water has been found to have a wildly variable amount of bacteria, while

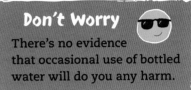

Don't Worry
There's no evidence that occasional use of bottled water will do you any harm.

tap water in wealthy industrialized nations has consistently low amounts. In the US, the EPA requires localities to regularly report on the health and safety of their tap water; no such rule exists for bottled water.

And yet the makers of bottled water have persuaded us to *pay them money* when a more healthy alternative literally flows into our sink.

STEP 1: Have some bottled water on hand in case of emergency.

STEP 2: If you're someplace without access to properly treated tap water, go ahead and drink bottled water without worrying about it.

STEP 3: If local health authorities recommend filtering your tap water, get the appropriate kind of filter.

STEP 4: Otherwise, unless you have specific evidence to the contrary, assume your tap water is healthier than bottled.

☐ If you've drunk tap water instead of bottled water, give yourself the win.

AVOID BAD FATS

Fat is good for you! It provides energy, helps you absorb vitamins, and improves your heart health.

Also, fat is bad for you! It raises cholesterol and makes your heart less healthy.

That paradox has a simple explanation: There are different kinds of fat.

Good Fats

Omega-3 fats can help reduce your risk of heart disease.

Good sources of omega-3 fats:

- Salmon, mackerel, albacore tuna, sardines, and other fatty fish
- Soybean products like tofu
- Walnuts
- Flaxseed
- Canola oil

Monounsaturated and polyunsaturated fat can improve your cholesterol.

Good sources of these fats include:

- Olive oil and olives
- Almonds, cashews, pine nuts, and many other nuts and seeds
- Avocados
- Vegetable oils

Bad Fats

Most animal fats are saturated fats. They increase your level of bad LDL cholesterol.

Sources of saturated fats include:

- Fatty cuts of meat
- Whole-fat dairy products like cheese, butter, whole milk, and cream
- Palm and coconut oils

Trans fats are mostly found in processed foods. They don't just increase your bad LDL cholesterol—they simultaneously lower your good HDL cholesterol.

Sources of trans fats include:

- Anything with "partially hydrogenated" oils listed in the ingredients
- Many prepackaged sweets and snacks

STEP 1: Next time you're tempted to eat a food with bad fat, see if you can substitute one with good fat (or at least less fat). Here are some ideas.

INSTEAD OF . . .	TRY . . .
Spreading butter on your toast	Dipping your toast in extra-virgin olive oil
A slice of cheese on your sandwich	A slice of avocado
Whole milk	Skim or 2% milk
Pre-packaged microwave popcorn with partially hydrogenated oil	Freshly popped popcorn with canola oil

☐ If you've cut back on one source of trans fat or saturated fat, feast on a win.

MODERATE YOUR MEAT

I don't claim to know where souls come from, but if they're biological in origin, it seems to me that animals close to us on the evolutionary tree might have them. For that reason, I stopped eating my fellow mammals decades ago.

My philosophical quirkiness may end up saving my life. Red meat is associated with increased risk of colorectal cancer—in fact, with a shorter lifespan in general. Processed red meat, like bacon and sausages, may be the worst of all.

To be clear, processed white meat is linked with colorectal cancer risk as well; my conscience may be untroubled by the chicken sausage and turkey bacon I've eaten, but my colon may well regret it. That's something I only learned in writing this book, and moving forward, I'll take my poultry unprocessed. So if find yourself missing the salty crunch of bacon...well, my friend, I feel your pain.

STEP 1: Consider how much processed meat and unprocessed red meat you typically eat.

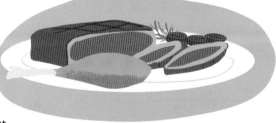

STEP 2: Try to substitute chicken or seafood for at least some of the red meat.

STEP 3: When you do have red meat, have it in as unprocessed a form as possible. A steak or spare rib is less likely to cause cancer than bacon or sausage.

☐ If you cut back on the amount of red meat in your diet (processed or unprocessed), bite into a thick, juicy win.

STOP DRINKING SUGAR

Sweetened drinks are the number one source of added sugar in many people's diets. On the plus side, that means most people can instantly make their diets healthier by modifying what they drink.

STEP 1: Don't try to go cold turkey. Put a little less sugar in your tea or coffee every day to help you get used to the taste. You can even try gradually watering down your sodas.

STEP 2: Drink more water. If you don't like the taste of water, try putting a slice of fruit in it. Or spring for sugar-free fizzy water.

STEP 3: For a sweet treat, pop some fruits and veggies into a blender with plain low-fat yogurt or water and make a healthy, homemade smoothie.

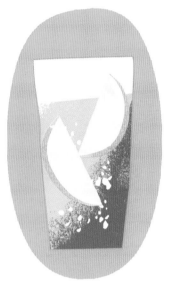

☐ If you've cut back on the amount of sugar you drink—even by a tiny amount—guzzle down the win.

WATCH THE BOOZE

After a few years of confusing headlines in the popular press, medical science seems to have settled into a clear view on alcohol:

If you don't drink, doctors wouldn't advise you to start, because too much alcohol increases your risk of dementia, and even light drinking increases your risk of cancer. If you do drink, doctors encourage you to sip heart-healthy red wine rather than caloric beer.

What Is a Unit?

Step 2 tells you how many drinks per week you should consume. There's just one question: What's a drink?

The National Institute of Health defines a "standard drink" as 0.6 fluid ounces or 14 grams of pure alcohol. Since some liquids are more alcoholic than others, how much beverage you have to consume to get those 14 grams will vary.

So, in practice, one drink is . . .

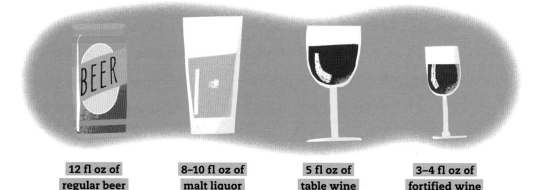

| 12 fl oz of regular beer | 8–10 fl oz of malt liquor | 5 fl oz of table wine | 3–4 fl oz of fortified wine |

STEP 1: If you don't drink alcohol, there's no need to start. You also shouldn't drink if you're pregnant, on any medication that could interact with alcohol, or planning on driving.

STEP 2: If you do drink, stop at two drinks a day for men, or one drink a day for women. Note that you can stop well before you reach that limit! Less alcohol is better than more.

STEP 3: To translate "drinks" into something more intuitive, see how many ounces that would be of your favorite beverage. If you don't naturally think in ounces, bust out the measuring cup.

STEP 4: If you find yourself unable to stick within the recommended guidelines for alcohol (or if you have other concerns around drinking), contact your local Alcoholics Anonymous, or seek other professional help (page 4).

☐ If you stayed under the recommended guidelines, raise your moderately filled glass in triumph.

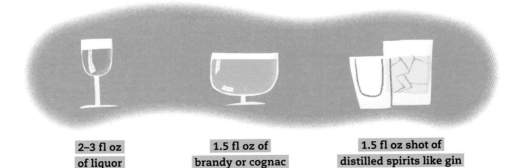

2–3 fl oz of liquor

1.5 fl oz of brandy or cognac

1.5 fl oz shot of distilled spirits like gin

CAFFEINATE

As the author of a book on better health, I am sometimes called upon to deliver bad news about your favorite vices. I am happy to report that at least one common vice is secretly a virtue:

Caffeine.

At least, caffeine in the form of coffee and green tea. Their mix of caffeine, antioxidants, and other nutrients may help prevent diabetes, cardiovascular disease, dementia, Parkinson's, and certain forms of cancer.

The evidence suggests that black tea has some, but not all, of its green cousin's disease-fighting power. But you don't get any benefits from a healthy beverage you refuse to drink. If green isn't your cup of tea, then feel free to enjoy black.

Everything has a downside. Coffee (especially unfiltered coffee) may increase bad cholesterol. Too much caffeine can raise your blood pressure. But up to around five cups of coffee or tea a day, the evidence suggests that you're doing more good than harm.

STEP 1: If you get your buzz from soda, switch over to coffee or tea. One cup of green tea has about as much caffeine as a twelve-ounce can of Coke—but the Coke has a whopping nine teaspoons of sugar, while the tea has none. If you can't quit sugar cold turkey, switch from soda to sweetened tea or coffee. Then go to Step 3.

. . . .

STEP 2: If you like tea or coffee without sugar, high-fat milk, or cream, go ahead and enjoy two to five cups a day.

. . . .

STEP 3: If you are used to adding sugar, cream, or high-fat milk to your brew, wean yourself gradually by adding a little less every day. If you don't like the resulting flavor, you can mellow your drink with skim or semi-skim milk. (Pro tip: A home milk foamer can make even skim milk feel fancy.)

STEP 4: Remember that caffeine has a half-life of five hours. If you drink two cups of coffee at 5 PM, you'll have a full cup's worth of caffeine running through your veins at 10 PM. The American Academy of Sleep Medicine recommends that you don't have any caffeine at all within six hours of bedtime.

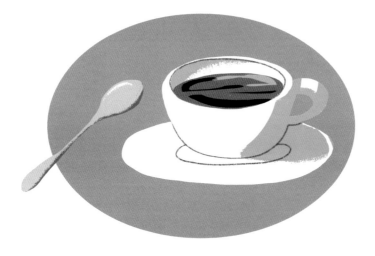

☐ If you've had one cup of tea or coffee without added sugar, feel the buzz.

DON'T SWEAT HYDRATION

Looking after your health can feel like running on a treadmill, even when you aren't actually running on a treadmill. As soon as you think you're doing enough, somebody comes along with a new rule to follow.

Well, I'm pleased to tell you there is one rule you don't need to worry about: You don't actually need to drink eight glasses of pure water every day.

Sure, most people need sixty ounces of water a day. But we can get it from a variety of sources. Healthy beverages like coffee, tea, and low-fat milk are mostly water, and so are many foods. For that matter, so are unhealthy beverages like sugary soda and alcohol (but see pages 99 and 100 before you start guzzling Coke and booze like water).

For example, apples are 85 percent water; coffee is 98 percent. If you start your day with a single apple and a cup of coffee, you've had nine or ten fluid ounces of water before you've had a single glass of pure H_2O.

STEP 1: Eat a variety of fruits and vegetables.

STEP 2: Drink healthy beverages when you're thirsty.

STEP 3: If you're not sure you're properly hydrated, try the pee test on page 105.

STEP 4: Unless you've got medical advice to the contrary, don't bother counting cups of water.

> If you've kept yourself hydrated (even if you didn't drink a full eight cups of water), drink in the win.

PEER AT YOUR PEE

Sometimes you get so dehydrated that the person you're with transforms into a giant bottle of fizzy water. (I usually get my scientific information from peer-reviewed journals, but occasionally I turn to Bugs Bunny cartoons.)

Other times, the signs are more subtle. If you keep an eye out for those signs, you can catch dehydration earlier, before it leads to headaches, confusion, or pulling on Daffy's head as if it were a bottle top.

One of the best signs is your own thirst. As in so many things, if you listen to your own body, you're likely to be fine. But there are exceptions. Being in an unfamiliar climate or doing more exercise than you're used to can throw off your bodily perceptions. And then there's the simple act of aging; older people may be less sensitive to thirst.

If you want to check your internal sensations against some external evidence, and you don't mind peering at your own pee, try this test.

STEP 1: Before you urinate, make sure the bowl has been flushed.

STEP 2: Pee.

STEP 3: Compare the color of your pee to this chart. If your urine is completely clear and colorless, you may be drinking too much water. If your urine is too dark, you need to drink more water.

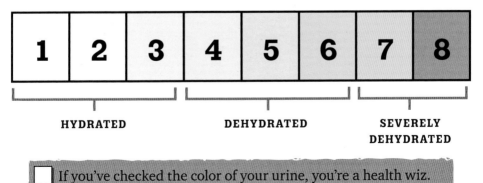

| 1 | 2 | 3 | 4 | 5 | 6 | 7 | 8 |

HYDRATED   DEHYDRATED   SEVERELY
                                      DEHYDRATED

☐ If you've checked the color of your urine, you're a health wiz.

HAVE A LITTLE CHOCOLATE

Good news: Dark chocolate may reduce your risk of stroke, heart disease, diabetes, and cancer!

Bad news: The evidence is not yet conclusive. And if there is a benefit, it probably comes from small amounts of chocolate. Eat too much, and the harm of the fat and sugar will outweigh the benefits of the cacao.

In short, don't consider this a license to camp out in the candy aisle. If you are the rare human who doesn't enjoy chocolate, don't force yourself to eat it. But if you enjoy chocolate in moderation, it may do you some good.

STEP 1: Get some dark chocolate. If you're going strictly for health purposes, you won't eat much of it, so get the best quality stuff you can afford. In my experience, a small square of fantastic chocolate is at least as satisfying as a big bar of the cheap stuff.

STEP 2: Measure 1.6 ounces of it. If you don't have a kitchen scale, you can just break off about a third of a standard 3.5-ounce chocolate bar.

STEP 3: Eat it slowly, savoring it.

SNAP! *SNAP!* *SNAP!*

If you've enjoyed a small amount of dark chocolate, you don't need me to tell you that's a win.

GO NUTS

Healthy doesn't always mean convenient. Fruits and vegetables have to be washed or chopped or refrigerated or cooked or some combination. It's no wonder we turn to ultra-processed snack foods (page 80).

If you want a convenient, portable snack that's healthy in moderation . . . it's nuts to the rescue!

Nuts are high in fiber and protein, and low in unhealthy saturated fatty acids. And if you eat a variety of them, you'll get a variety of beneficial nutrients. Brazil nuts and almonds are high in magnesium. Pistachios brim with potassium. Macadamias give you lots of zinc.

Nuts are also high in calories, so you probably shouldn't eat them for breakfast, lunch, and dinner. But they are a definite part of a healthy snack portfolio.

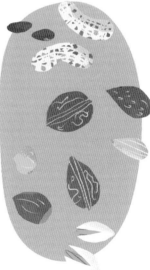

STEP 1: If you're in a shared environment, make sure nobody around you has a nut allergy.

. . . .

STEP 2: Have shelled, unsalted nuts on hand. (Technically, peanuts are legume seeds rather than nuts—but they're as crunchy and healthy as true nuts, so feel free to include them.)

. . . .

STEP 3: When you want a convenient, crunchy snack, grab a handful.

☐ If you've eaten one serving of nuts, go nuts.

EAT A SINGLE RAISIN

This tip, and the next two, involves **mindful eating**. Think of mindful eating as meditation at the dinner table. It involves being present and aware, in a nonjudgmental way, as you eat.

Mindful eating may be as effective a short-term weight-loss tool as a diet. In the long term, alas, diets don't work (page 81). Does mindful eating fare better? I haven't yet seen any studies that answer that.

At the very least, you'll probably enjoy your meals more if you notice the taste. And introducing mindfulness at the table may help you be more present and calm in your daily life.

One way to start is with this simple exercise, popularized by mindfulness expert Jon Kabat-Zinn.

STEP 1: Get a single raisin. Put it in front of you. (If you can't stand raisins, you can use a single grape, or a nut, or any other healthy food you enjoy.)

STEP 2: Before you taste it, experience it with your other senses. Smell it. Roll it around your fingers. Look at it closely. Hold it up to your ear and squish it. You're not trying to come to any particular conclusion; you're just observing.

STEP 3: Now put the raisin in your mouth. Let it rest on your tongue. What does it taste and feel like?

STEP 4: Start chewing as slowly as you can. How does the flavor and texture change as you bite into it?

STEP 5: When it is completely chewed, swallow it. Close your eyes, and savor the aftertaste.

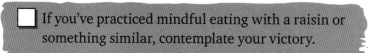

☐ If you've practiced mindful eating with a raisin or something similar, contemplate your victory.

PERFORM A PREMEAL WARM-UP

Checking in with yourself before you pop that snack into your mouth can help make sure you're eating because you're hungry and not because you're bored or frustrated.

This warm-up is based on one from Dr. Judson Brewer, an addiction psychologist.

STEP 1: Before you eat, check in with your body. How hungry are you on a scale of zero to ten, where zero is "utterly famished" and ten is "just finished Thanksgiving dinner and can't move from the couch"?

STEP 2: Before you taste the food, give two other senses a workout. How does it look? What does it smell like?

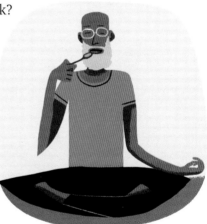

STEP 3: Take a single bite. Pay attention to the food's taste and mouthfeel.

STEP 4: Check in with your body again. Still hungry?

> ☐ If you've performed a premeal warm-up before your most recent meal, warm up to a win.

PUT DOWN THE FORK

In high school, I had a short lunch period. With grace beforehand and post-lunch announcements afterward, the actual eating time was even shorter, and I got into the habit of shoveling food into my mouth as if it were an Olympic sport.

Decades later, I still sometimes find myself wolfing down my grub like a rushed teenager. A simple exercise has helped me eat more mindfully. That makes me much less likely to keep eating past the point of satiety—and it makes things taste better, too.

STEP 1: After you put food into your mouth, put the fork down on the table and let go of it.

STEP 2: Don't pick it up until you've chewed and swallowed the food already in your mouth.

STEP 3: If you're eating finger food, don't pick up the next bite until you've completely finished the current one.

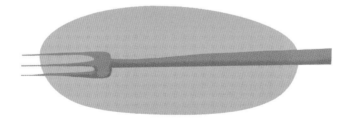

If you've put the fork down between bites, pick up a win.

TREAT FOOD LIKE AN EXPERIMENT

The snack food industry spends billions of dollars every year on research and development. It's no coincidence that unhealthy foods taste so good.

If you want healthy food to compete on flavor, you're going to have to be your own research scientist.

STEP 1: Take a fruit or vegetable you like. If you're a die-hard produce hater, take the one you dislike the least.

STEP 2: Prepare it two ways—raw versus cooked, or steamed versus sauteed, or as part of two different stews.

STEP 3: Don't add too many unhealthy ingredients—if you're comparing "apples served with a bowlful of potato chips" versus "apples served with a tablespoon of sugar," you're missing the point.

STEP 4: Taste both versions. Which one do you like better? Are there elements of both you might want to combine?

STEP 5: Use what you've learned to search for two new recipes. If you liked the sauteed broccoli better than steamed, search the internet for "sauteed broccoli recipes."

STEP 6: Make both new recipes and compare them.

STEP 7: Keep repeating the process until you've got a dish that's as addictive as an ultra-processed shelf-stable food product, but a million times healthier.

☐ If you've compared two recipes, you're a comparative winner.

EAT THE RAINBOW

It's important to eat a wide variety of fruits and vegetables, because each one has a different balance of nutrients. Blueberries have healthy antioxidants called anthocyanins. Spinach is rich in the essential nutrient folate.

And you know what? Ten seconds after you read that paragraph, you're likely to forget it. I've forgotten what blueberries have, ten seconds after I *wrote* it.

Fortunately, if you don't want to memorize the nutritional benefits of every fruit or vegetable in the world, you can fall back on an easy rule of thumb: Different-colored produce is likely to be rich in different nutrients.

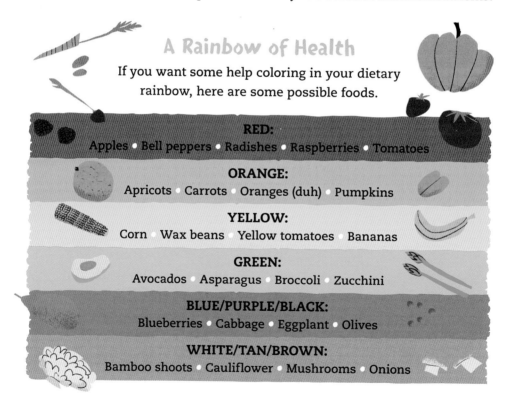

A Rainbow of Health

If you want some help coloring in your dietary rainbow, here are some possible foods.

RED:
Apples • Bell peppers • Radishes • Raspberries • Tomatoes

ORANGE:
Apricots • Carrots • Oranges (duh) • Pumpkins

YELLOW:
Corn • Wax beans • Yellow tomatoes • Bananas

GREEN:
Avocados • Asparagus • Broccoli • Zucchini

BLUE/PURPLE/BLACK:
Blueberries • Cabbage • Eggplant • Olives

WHITE/TAN/BROWN:
Bamboo shoots • Cauliflower • Mushrooms • Onions

STEP 1: Eat one serving of a fruit or vegetable.

STEP 2: At some point in the day, try to eat a fruit or vegetable that's a different color.

STEP 3: Aim to eat all the colors of the rainbow every day.

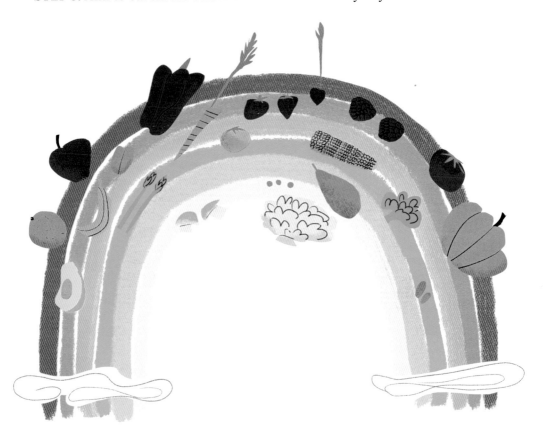

☐ If you've eaten the rainbow today, give yourself a colorful win.

EAT SEASONALLY

If you don't like healthy food, I'm with you. I hate strawberries. They're tasteless, watery things...in winter. But in spring? Oh my God. They are so sweet and fragrant that I feel like I'm getting away with something: *Are you telling me that this deliciousness is* **good for me???**

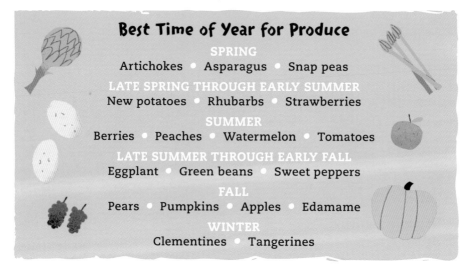

Best Time of Year for Produce

SPRING
Artichokes • Asparagus • Snap peas

LATE SPRING THROUGH EARLY SUMMER
New potatoes • Rhubarbs • Strawberries

SUMMER
Berries • Peaches • Watermelon • Tomatoes

LATE SUMMER THROUGH EARLY FALL
Eggplant • Green beans • Sweet peppers

FALL
Pears • Pumpkins • Apples • Edamame

WINTER
Clementines • Tangerines

STEP 1: Look up the peak season for various fruits and vegetables—even ones you think you don't like. The box above will give you a general idea, although the actual months may vary depending on where you live. Try searching the web for "rhubarb season in South US," or whatever combination of produce and geography applies to you.

STEP 2: Mark your calendar for the year ahead with produce you want to try.

STEP 3: Buy fresh fruits and vegetables at the right time of year, and see if the flavor was worth waiting for.

☐ If you've eaten seasonal produce, it's the right time for a win.

EAT LOCALLY

The faster fruits and vegetables reach your plate, the more nutrients they retain. A head of broccoli that was picked yesterday has more vitamin C than one that was picked two weeks ago.

Alas, unless the farmer is a former librarian who stamps the date on every cucumber, you can't know exactly when it was picked. But you do know this: Transporting food takes time. All things being equal, a tomato that was grown down the block is probably fresher than one from the other side of the world.

As a bonus, local vegetables often taste better. A farmer whose apples are going to travel thousands of miles has to breed them for hardiness; a farmer who is selling them in a local market can breed them purely on taste.

Don't Worry

Local, seasonal produce may be the most healthy, but store-bought fruits and vegetables are still plenty good for you.

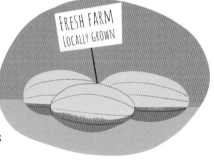

STEP 1: Find a farmers market in your area. Ask around, or type "local farmers market" in your search engine of choice.

STEP 2: Visit the farmers market. If you're not sure what to buy, ask the people who grew it. One of the benefits of a farmers market is that you get direct access to their expertise.

STEP 3: Alternatively, search for "CSA" or "community supported agriculture." With a CSA, you pay a local farmer in advance, and then you get a share of everything they grow that season.

STEP 4: Enjoy your healthy, delicious locally grown produce.

☐ If you've purchased or eaten locally grown produce, harvest your win.

FREEZE!

Which is healthier: fresh vegetables or frozen?

The answer is more complicated than you think. Freezing usually occurs soon after harvest, which helps preserve nutrients. Hooray! But before they're frozen, fruits and vegetables are often blanched (heated quickly at a high temperature), which can destroy nutrients. Boo! But because they've been blanched, you don't have to heat them as much at home, which helps preserve nutrients. Hooray!

All in all, by the time those peas journey from the ground to your mouth, frozen is probably as good as fresh. Canned produce may lose more nutrients than frozen, but it's still better than nothing. Plus, it's good to eat a rainbow of fruits and vegetables (page 112), and a well-stocked freezer and pantry makes that easier.

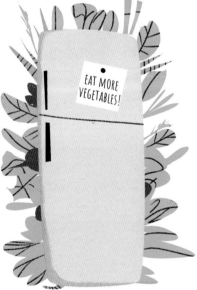

EAT MORE VEGETABLES!

STEP 1: If you enjoy a fruit or vegetable you can't buy locally (or if you want to store it for a long time), consider buying it frozen or canned.

STEP 2: Before you buy, check the ingredients. Ideally, the only thing listed will be the fruit or vegetable itself. Avoid sugar and salt as much as possible. And skip ultra-processed vegetables entirely (page 80).

☐ If you've stored produce in the fridge or freezer, enjoy an ice-cold victory.

COMPARE APPLES TO APPLES

I love apples, but I don't like apples, and I think apples are just so-so.

If that doesn't make sense, let me be more specific: I love Gala apples, but I don't like Braeburn apples, and I think Red Delicious apples are just so-so.

If you've tried a fruit or vegetable and haven't enjoyed it, the problem could be the variety. And if you do enjoy it, you might find a variety you like even more.

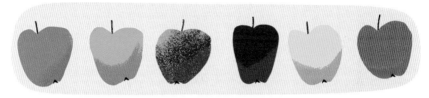

STEP 1: Find a fruit or vegetable you like. Buy as many different varieties as you can.

STEP 2: Do a taste test and see which one you like best.

STEP 3: Repeat the process, but with a fruit or vegetable you don't like. You might end up adding a new favorite to your repertoire.

STEP 4: This works for healthy beverages, too. If you're trying to switch from soda to tea, you might find you like Japanese sencha more than English breakfast.

STEP 5: If you buy from somebody who knows their stuff, tell them what you're looking for and see if they have advice. At my local farmers market, I can tell the apple grower, "I want something as fragrant as a Cox but less tart," and he'll know exactly what to suggest.

☐ If you've tried two varieties of the same fruit or vegetable, give yourself one variety of victory.

TAKE YOUR VITAMINS—BUT DON'T TAKE THEM TOO FAR

Vitamin supplements will result in healthier joints, clearer skin, and faster brains . . . or so vitamin manufacturers claim.

But if you ask doctors—whose incentive is to keep you healthy, not to sell you things—they'll say that vitamins mostly give you expensive urine. Eating a balanced and healthy diet gives you most of the nutrients you need. Anything extra you take in pill form is just going to come out the other end.

There are a few exceptions to the Get Your Vitamins from Food rule:

- **Your body needs sunlight to make vitamin D, and if you don't live close to the equator, there may be times of year when sunlight is in short supply.**

- **Anyone who is pregnant (or trying to get there) can benefit from taking folic acid, which helps prevent birth defects like spina bifida.**

STEP 1: If you're pregnant, or might become pregnant, take a folic acid supplement. The CDC recommends four hundred micrograms of folic acid every day.

STEP 2: The amount of vitamin D you need in pill form can vary depending on how old you are, how far you live from the equator, and how many vitamin D–enriched foods you eat. According to the NIH, most adults need a total of fifteen micrograms from diet and pills combined. You can ask your doctor for more personalized advice.

STEP 3: If your doctor has told you to take any other vitamins, follow their expert advice. Otherwise, save your money.

☐ If you took vitamin D, or stopped taking other vitamins unnecessarily, take your daily win.

HEALTHY
ALL OVER

There's more to fitness than just eating right and exercising. There are roughly 37,200,000,000,000 cells in your body, and every one of them deserves love and care.

OPEN A WINDOW

I just checked out your home, and I've got bad news for you.

You've got a high concentration of carbon dioxide, which causes drowsiness and confusion. You've got lots of humidity, which encourages mold growth. And if you've got more than one person inside, you're constantly breathing in each other's germs.

But don't worry! You can flush your home with a healthy mixture of nitrogen, oxygen, and other gases just by following my patented three-step process!

STEP 1: Open a window.

STEP 2: If you've got another window, open it as well, to get a cross-breeze.

STEP 3: If you live in an area with bad air pollution, you might want to open your windows at night, when pollution tends to be better, then close them during the day. Or open them in bursts, then close them and run an air filter (page 121).

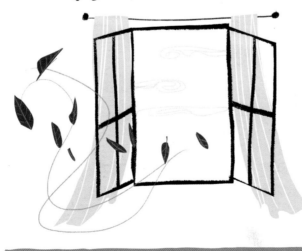

If you opened your window today, breathe in the win.

GET AN AIR FILTER

Air pollution kills 8.8 million people a year. If it doesn't kill you, it can make you stupid—among its many other consequences, air pollution lowers cognitive ability.

So while you've got some brain cells left, do the smart thing: Protect yourself.

STEP 1: Visit **airnow.gov**, and check your local air quality. If it's bad, close your windows and run an air filter.

STEP 2: If you have to be outside in a polluted area (or if you're biking along a busy roadway), wear a mask. You'll filter out the most pollution with a dust respirator or a Teflon filter, but a surgical face mask will still filter out about 80 percent of the pollutants. Even a handkerchief wrapped around your head is better than nothing.

STEP 3: Encourage your elected officials to treat pollution as the serious public health issue that it is.

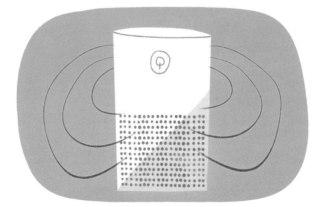

☐ If you've taken steps to protect yourself from air pollution, breathe in some fresh victory.

GET CHECKED

Figuring out which checkups you need is surprisingly complex. For example, if you have a prostate, should you be screened for prostate cancer? That depends, among other things, on your age, your ethnicity, your own medical history, and your family medical history. I could make a chapter-length flow chart for that one specific test, and it still wouldn't capture the expertise stored in your doctor's noggin.

So what follows is a rough guide to the average frequency of some commonly needed checkups. Even that is subject to caveats and variations. View it as a starting point for a conversation with your medical professional.

How Often to Get Checked

See your . . .
- **Dentist:** Once or twice a year
- **Doctor:** As often as your doctor recommends

Get a . . .
- **Eye exam:** Every two years after the age of forty if you're Black (after the age of sixty if you aren't)
- **Pap smear for sexually active people with cervixes:** Every three years until you turn sixty-five

Get screened for . . .
- **High blood pressure:** Annually for anybody forty years or older and for adults who are Black, overweight or obese, or otherwise at increased risk. For other adults aged eighteen to thirty-nine years, every three to five years.
- **Colorectal cancer:** After the age of forty-five (how often depends on the specific test)

STEP 1: If you're overdue for anything on the "Get Checked" list, make an appointment.

STEP 2: Remember: This list is for people who aren't showing symptoms of any medical problems. If you're having trouble seeing, it doesn't matter how old you are or when you last had an eye exam. Book an appointment now.

STEP 3: Any time you visit a health-care professional, ask when you should next see them, and if there are any other tests or appointments you should have in the meantime.

STEP 4: Make the appointment. Mark the date in your calendar, set your phone to remind you, or do whatever else you need to make sure you show up.

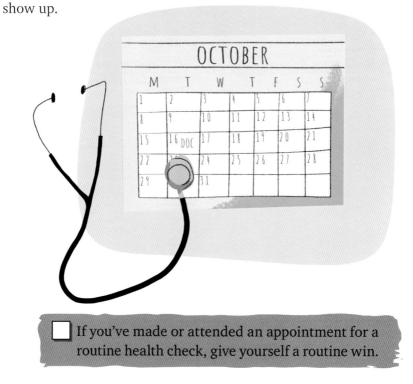

☐ If you've made or attended an appointment for a routine health check, give yourself a routine win.

TREAT YOUR CHOMPERS WELL

Brushing your teeth is something most of us learn how to do in childhood—but surprisingly few of us learned it right.

STEP 1: Brush your teeth once before bed, and one other time during the day. Your toothbrush should have soft bristles and be no more than three or four months old. Replace it sooner if the bristles get worn down.

STEP 2: Use a fluoride toothpaste. You just need a pea-size amount—those giant slugs of toothpaste you see in ads are just there to show off the product.

STEP 3: Place your toothbrush at a forty-five-degree angle to the gums. You want the tips of the bristles to slide under the gumline and clean out any nasties lurking there.

STEP 4: Move the brush back and forth with short strokes, as if you're polishing each tooth. Don't push too hard. If you want a sense of how gentle brushing should be, hold an orange in your hand. The pressure it makes on your hand is about how hard you should push on your teeth. (Alternatively, many electric toothbrushes have sensors to warn you if you're pushing too hard.)

STEP 5: To clean inside your mouth, hold the toothbrush up or down, and make several up and down strokes.

STEP 6: Make sure you clean the tops of your teeth—the part you actually chew with.

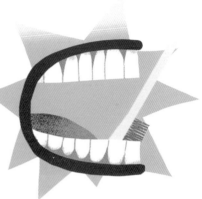

STEP 7: Brush for two minutes. If you go longer, you aren't providing any additional benefit, and you may irritate your gums.

STEP 8: When you finish, spit out the excess toothpaste, but don't rinse your mouth out. You've just applied cavity-preventing fluoride. The longer you let it linger, the better it can do its job.

STEP 9: Clean between your teeth once a day. Inter-dental brushes are better than dental floss. But not every inter-dental brush is right for every mouth, so ask your dentist for a recommendation. In the meantime, dental floss is better than nothing. It doesn't remove plaque as effectively as an inter-dental brush, but it can still reduce your risk of gingivitis (a fancy word for "inflamed gums").

☐ If you've cleaned your teeth properly, bite into a win.

CARE FOR YOUR BIGGEST ORGAN

Your skin is your biggest organ. It's also one of the few you can directly take care of.

These tips are courtesy of the American Academy of Dermatology.

STEP 1: Apply moisturizer when your skin is damp so that it can trap the moisture inside. Keep hand cream next to your soap, and use it every time you wash your hands.

STEP 2: Limit face washing to twice a day and after sweating. Apply gentle, alcohol-free cleanser with your fingertips, and use lukewarm water. For the skin under your eyes, use your ring finger; it's the weakest finger, and therefore the least likely to pull on that sensitive spot. Pat dry with a soft towel.

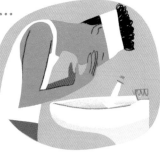

STEP 3: Ironically, too many antiaging products can irritate your skin, making the signs of aging more visible. If you're moisturizing your skin and protecting it from the sun (page 127), you may already be doing enough. If you're still concerned about aging, consider using retinol or another retinoid—but check with your doctor or dermatologist first. Retinoids shouldn't be used during pregnancy, and they aren't suitable for every skin type.

STEP 4: Look at your skin regularly over your entire body. Use a mirror to examine body parts you can't otherwise see. If you notice changes, speak to your doctor. Skin cancer is highly treatable if it's caught early enough.

☐ If you've taken one step to care for your largest organ, give yourself the biggest win.

FIGHT THE SUN

You versus the sun. It doesn't sound like a fair fight, does it? Your foe has 1.9885×10^{30} kilograms of flaming gas. What have you got?

You've got *science*. And it's going to help you avoid skin cancer, sunburns, and visible signs of aging, if only you'll listen to it.

STEP 1: Search online for "UV index" plus the name of your area to find a forecast for how strong the sun's UV rays will be. If it's going to be three or higher, take steps to protect your skin and eyes. Specifically . . .

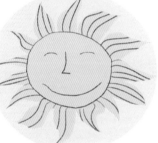

STEP 2: Slather on the sunscreen (SPF 15 or higher). If you're in the sun for more than two hours, reapply it.

STEP 3: Wear sunglasses and a broad-brimmed hat. Make sure your sunglasses block both UVA and UVB light. Wraparound sunglasses offer additional protection against sneaky sunbeams creeping in from the sides.

STEP 4: Sunscreen is great protection, but it's not perfect. Even when you're wearing it, seek out natural shade as much as possible, and try to avoid being outside during the peak UV times of day. In most places, this is between roughly 10 AM and 4 PM.

STEP 5: Spending a sunny day at the beach? Wear sunscreen even on parts of your body that will be covered by cloth. (And remember: Wet clothes offer less UV protection than dry ones.) Don't forget to reapply sunscreen after swimming.

☐ If you've taken one step to protect your skin and eyes against UV rays, wear a sunny smile.

GIVE BLOOD

One blood donation can save up to three lives. Four, if you include a life that may be of some importance to you: your own. People who donate regularly may have reduced risk of cancer and heart attack. Scientists are still figuring out why, but they think donating blood may prevent you from having too much iron in your system.

Sometimes you have to choose between helping other people and helping yourself. Blood donation is a rare opportunity to do both.

STEP 1: Look up your local blood donation center.

....

STEP 2: Make an appointment to give blood.

....

STEP 3: Show up and save somebody else's life while extending your own.

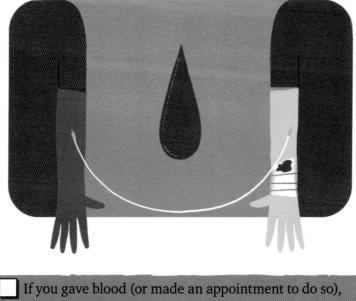

☐ If you gave blood (or made an appointment to do so), donate a win to yourself.

OVER THE LIPS AND PAST THE TEETH

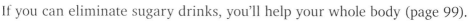

If you can eliminate sugary drinks, you'll help your whole body (page 99). In the meantime, you can help your teeth by using a straw. It's a simple step that will reduce the contact between the enamel that protects your teeth and the sugar that eats away at it. The same goes for acidic beverages (which includes most fizzy drinks).

> **Don't Worry**
>
> No one drink is going to do much harm. This tip is meant to avoid cumulative damage over a lifetime of sips.

STEP 1: Next time you drink something sweet, acidic, or fizzy, use a straw.

STEP 2: If you drink a lot of these beverages, help the environment by carrying a reusable straw.

STEP 3: If you can, have your tooth-damaging drink with a meal. Food will help reduce the harm done by your beverage.

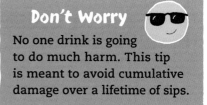

☐ If you took one step to prevent a beverage from harming your teeth, slurp up a victory.

PROTECT YOUR EARS

Your ears are a miracle of biological engineering. Within each one, an elaborately shaped piece of skin and cartilage funnels energy waves toward a flexible membrane that vibrates the three smallest bones in your body, thereby transmitting the waves through a fluid that triggers twenty-five thousand nerve endings, which convert them into electrical impulses, which your brain interprets as music or language or claps of thunder.

It's a complex and delicate system. One of the most important things you can do to keep it working is to avoid exposure to loud noises.

If you've got a smartphone, download the NIOSH Sound Level Meter, or whatever sound meter app you can find for your platform. It won't be as accurate as a professionally calibrated sound meter, but it will give you a sense of the volume levels in your everyday life. Otherwise, a rough rule of thumb is this:

If the noise is loud enough to drown out a normal speaking voice, take steps to protect your hearing.

Noise Levels

NOISE	TYPICAL DECIBEL LEVEL	TYPICAL NEGATIVE EFFECT
Normal conversation	60 dB	None
Washing machine; dishwasher	70 dB	Annoyance
Gas-powered lawnmower; leaf blower	80-85 dB	Hearing damage possible after 2 hours of exposure
Motorcycle	95 dB	Hearing damage possible after 50 minutes of exposure
Sporting event; oncoming subway train	100 dB	Hearing loss possible after 15 minutes
Rock concert; a personal listening device set at maximum volume	105-110 dB	Hearing loss possible in less than 5 minutes
Standing beside or near sirens	120 dB	Pain and ear injury
Firecrackers	140-150 dB	Pain and ear injury

STEP 1: If you'll be someplace with dangerous volume levels, take earplugs or noise-canceling headphones. Wear them as soon as the noise starts. I keep a pair of foam earplugs tucked inside my glasses case.

STEP 2: If you go to a lot of concerts, look into getting earplugs designed specifically for music. They protect your ears without ruining the tune.

STEP 3: If you are in a noisy place and don't have hearing protection, you have two options. There's a little flap of skin on your ear called the tragus, and you can push firmly on it to seal your ear canal. Or you can stick your fingers in your ears. There is some evidence that fingers-in-the-ears is the more effective of these two methods, but I couldn't find any definitive studies. Your best bet may be to get out of the noisy situation as soon as you can.

STEP 4: If you listen to music with headphones, see if your device has a built-in setting to prevent dangerously loud volumes. Otherwise, have somebody stand next to you while you listen at your usual level. If the bystander can hear your music, it's too loud.

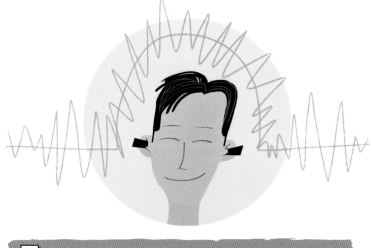

☐ If you've taken one step to protect your hearing, listen to the sound of victory.

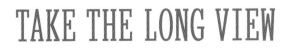

TAKE THE LONG VIEW

The average American worker spends about seven hours a day on the computer—and that doesn't include time spent staring at their phone. But keeping your eyes unceasingly focused on a constant near distance can cause **computer vision syndrome**, which can involve eye strain, headaches, blurred vision, or shoulder pain.

Next time your boss comes by and finds you staring idly out the window, tell them you're just following doctor's orders.

STEP 1: Set a reminder on your computer to take a break every twenty minutes.

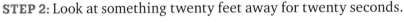

STEP 2: Look at something twenty feet away for twenty seconds.

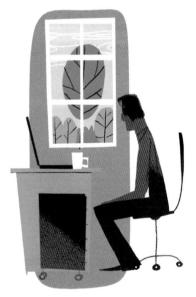

☐ If you've taken a break to look in the distance, gaze upon victory.

GO WITH YOUR GUT

If I were the only person on earth, I could still look in a mirror and say, "We need fiber to stay healthy."

I wouldn't be using the royal we. I would be referring to me and my gut biome—a collection of roughly 100 trillion helpful bacteria that live in my digestive system. Scientists are only beginning to discover what those teeny guys are up to, but they suspect it's lots of good things; healthy gut biomes have been implicated in preventing depression, fighting obesity, and preventing a whole host of illnesses.

Science Says No

Given where the science stands now, it's not worth buying expensive probiotic supplements. As with so many other allegedly miraculous pills, you're better off eating a healthy and varied diet.

STEP 1: Eat a "probiotic food"—one that has live, healthy bacteria in it. This includes many yogurts, sauerkrauts, and kombucha teas (although make sure the label says "live" or "active" bacteria; sometimes they are killed in the process of making the food).

STEP 2: Eat a "prebiotic food"— one that's rich in fiber that your biome will love. This includes foods like apples or Jerusalem artichokes.

☐ If you've eaten or drank something that's good for your biome, you know in your gut it's a win.

GIVE YOUR KNEES A BREAK

There's a myth that running wears down your knees, ultimately leading to arthritis. That doesn't seem to be true—but if your knees are aching for more than an hour after a workout, it may be a sign that you need to change something.

STEP 1: If your knees hurt after a workout, check the soles of your shoes. If they're worn down, it may be time to replace them. If you haven't had a professional shoe fitting recently, stop by a running or fitness store to make sure you've got the right shoes for you.

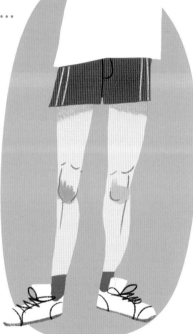

STEP 2: Consider switching to shorter but more frequent workouts. When you put stress on cartilage, it responds positively for the first ten minutes, undergoing changes that ultimately strengthen it. After that, you're not necessarily doing any long-term harm, but you're not getting any benefit, either.

STEP 3: Weeks or months before you start a more intense running routine or make any other change that will put extra strain on your knees, strengthen the muscles that support them. Do ten to fifteen lunges, rest for ten seconds, and then ten to fifteen squats. Repeat two or three more times.

☐ If you've taken steps to prevent knee pain, you've stepped toward victory.

HEALTHY SOUL

Quick. Off the top of your head, list the three best things you can do for your health. We'll say them together:

Quit smoking!

Take up exercise!

Play Dungeons and Dragons with your college roommate James!

Wait, you didn't say the last one? Maybe you should. According to a survey of 148 studies that collectively tracked 308,849 people across 7.5 years, having a strong social network improves your physical health as much as quitting smoking, and even *more* than exercise.

STEP 1: Reach out to a friend you already have. Texting, emailing, or calling all count, but a general post on social media doesn't; research has shown that direct personal contact is the best kind.

STEP 2: Look for opportunities to make new friends. Invite a coworker out for a coffee. Join a local chess club. Or, for a health boost that combines the physical and the social, join a local team (page 48).

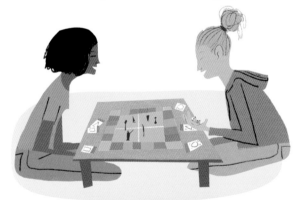

☐ If you've taken one step to form a new friendship or maintain an existing one, give yourself the win.

Acknowledgments

When I joined my high school swim team in my freshman year, I was the slowest kid on the team. I couldn't make it from one end of the pool to the other without grabbing onto the wall and catching my breath. By the time I graduated . . . well, I was still the slowest kid on the team. But I could swim the entire length of the pool without coming up for air, and then do a two-hour workout. I had learned from my coaches that it didn't matter how I compared with everybody else, as long as I did better than I did yesterday. Thank you to Coach Grant, Coach Green, and Coach Brockway for that lesson, which has served me just as well outside the pool as in it.

In 2019, my fantastic agent, Ammi-Joan Paquette, recognized that I'd click with the brilliant and passionate staff of Odd Dot and suggested that I stop by their offices and meet them. This is the fourth book to come out of that meeting. Thank you, Joan, for your ongoing insight and support.

And speaking of Odd Dot's brilliant and passionate staff, thank you to Nathalie Le Du, Christina Quintero, Kate Avino, Tim Hall, Caitlyn Hunter, Jen Healey, Barbara Cho, Kathy Wielgosz, and Tracy Koontz. I'm especially grateful to my editor Justin Krasner for trusting me with another book in the Be Better Now series.

Thank you Dr. Baturalp Baserdem for reading the manuscript with a medical professional's eye and letting me know what I got wrong. Needless to say, if I've persisted in any errors despite his thoughtful feedback, the responsibility is entirely mine.

A special thank you to my wife, Lauren, and my children, Erin and Joe, for their patience over the many days I hid away in my office to write this book, and their love and support always.